CONTENTS

INTRODUCTION

Indoor electric grills could easily be among everyone's favorite appliances of all time. Just imagine saying goodbye to the outdoors fuss and bringing the sunny grilling experience indoors not only during summer but all year round.

These kitchen gadgets come in two types: the contact grill and the open grill. The contact grill looks like a sandwich press that cooks food directly from two sides. The open grill, on the other hand, is similar to an electric griddle with ridges.

Indoor electric grills are not only popular during unfavorable weather conditions. These are also a big hit among those living in apartments and condominiums with limited space for grilling and entertaining a large group of visitors.

Using an indoor electric grill is also deemed safer and healthier as it eliminates the hazards of grilling outdoors, including burning coal, excessive smoke, and dripping fats.

With multifunctionality being a top trend in most kitchen gadgets in recent years, indoor electric grills can also do several things aside from yielding authentic char-grilled appearance, aroma, and taste in foods. Most indoor grills also function as another kitchen gadget craze—an air fryer. One such versatile kitchen appliance is the Ninja Foodi Smart XL Grill.

An Overview

What is the Ninja Foodi Smart XL Grill?

A 6-in-1 smokeless countertop grill, the Ninja Foodi Smart XL Grill can grill, air fry, bake, roast, broil and dehydrate foods. It comes with a 4-quart crisper basket and a 6-quart cooking pot. The air fry crisp function uses up to 75 percent less fat compared to deep frying.

Although this model cooks with its lid closed, only one side of food is in contact with the grill, making it an open grill type.

What are its Features and Functions?

The Ninja Foodi Smart XL Grill features a Smart Cook System and a 500-degree Cyclonic Grilling Technology for evenly cooked results.

Forget about second-guessing whether the food is undercooked or overcooked. With the Smart Cook System, a touch of a button is all it takes to get rare to well-done meat with char-grilled marks and flavors. It features a dual-sensor Foodi Smart Thermometer, four smart settings for protein, and nine doneness levels.

The 1,760-watt Ninja Foodi Smart XL Grill also boasts a smoke control system that effectively keeps smoke out of the kitchen. Coupled with a cool-air zone, it has a splatter shield and a temperature-regulating grill grate.

Perfect for family-sized meals, the XL capacity of this model translates to 50 percent more food than the original Ninja Foodi Grill version. The 9-by-12 inches grill grate can fit up to six steaks, 24 hotdogs, or a main and side dishes at the same time.

Tips for Getting Started

Using electric grills and air fryers can be intimidating if you are operating them for the first time. Fear not because we have curated a few tips that any beginner user should know. Read on and let us get you grilling and more in no time.

Always prioritize safety and set aside time for reading the user manual that comes along with the Ninja Foodie Smart XL Grill first.

Electric grills may not look like it, but they usually get hot during and after use. Practice caution and use safety tools such as tongs and oven mitts when handling the device and the food.

Place the grill on a heat-proof surface, leaving at least 5 inches of space on all sides for sufficient airflow. Also, do not place it near water to avoid electric shocks.

Allow the device to preheat for a few minutes before adding the food. Preheating will allow the grill to reach the right temperature that will give you evenly cooked and beautifully char-grilled results. Preheating also avoids extended cooking time and food from sticking to the grate.

Lightly grease the grill and basket even though they have nonstick coatings. Steer away, however, from aerosol cooking sprays as these can damage the device. We recommend getting a regular kitchen spray bottle filled with your choice of oil.

Cooking Tips & Tricks

The Ninja Foodi Smart XL Grill is practically like a convection oven. You can cook almost anything in it. You can use standard pans for baking with the air fryer function. From cakes and brownies to doughnuts and tarts--but keep an eye in case of the goods browning quickly.

You can also cook hard-boiled eggs directly in the air fryer. It would take about 15 minutes.

Try grilling vegetables such as broccoli wrapped in parchment paper. Doing so will give the vegetables the same texture from steaming, but with a hint of the charred flavor.

The air fryer is also perfect for toasting nuts. The cooking process will continue until after the nuts are unloaded from the fryer, so pull them out a bit earlier.

Frozen foods can also be cooked directly in your Ninja Foodi Smart XL Grill without thawing them first.

Say goodbye to bland and soggy leftovers—from roast chicken and salmon to pizza and vegetables. Reheat them in the air fryer for a crispier second time (or more) around.

Less is more when it comes to oil to achieve crispiness perfection. Grease too much, and you will get soggy instead of tasty evenly cooked crispy results. Neutral oils such as canola and vegetable oils are considered best for grilling because of their high smoking point. These also do not add unwanted flavor to the food.

Save the leftover fats in the pan for later to make pan sauces and gravies.

Even with its size, make it a habit to cook in batches with your Ninja Foodi Smart XL Grill. Overcrowding food tends to obscure the hot air circulation inside, thereby affecting the crispiness and doneness of the food. Larger meats like pork chops, chicken cutlets, steaks, burgers, and fish fillets should be arranged in a single layer and not stacked one on top of the other.

Shaking the basket from time to time will also help to make sure everything inside the basket will cook and brown evenly.

Use the Foodi Smart Thermometer to check the doneness of meat accurately. Doing so not only helps to prevent overcooking but also ensures that the food is cooked enough and safe to eat.

Use oil to weigh down and glue your seasonings to the food. The air circulation inside the appliance may blow off lightweight particles such as spices while cooking. You can avoid this by mixing spices with oil before coating the food with them.

When cooking with marinated meats, let them sit on a cooling rack first to drain the excess liquids. Unlike outdoor grills, indoor grills do not drain liquid as well. So, doing this extra step will save you from cleaning marinades that dripped over your counter.

Care & Maintenance Tips

With proper care and regular maintenance, your electric grill will surely last for years or even a lifetime. It is essential to clean the unit, not only to keep it running in tiptop shape but also for food safety reasons.

A sure sign that your electric grill needs some cleaning is when you start noticing smoke coming out of the machine while cooking. It signals an oil buildup. But cleaning an electric grill is so straightforward, you don't have to wait until the smoke detector alarms before taking action.

Cleaning the grill daily or after each use will avoid the accumulation of food residues in the grill. Make sure the device is turned off and unplugged, and let it cool down for a few minutes. It would be easier to clean the grate while it is still a bit hot, so take caution.

The machine itself, the basket, and the drip drawer will need a thorough cleaning. The detachable parts are dishwasher-safe, but the appliance itself is not.

The Ninja Foodi Smart XL Grill comes with a cleaning brush that you can use to get rid of the food leftovers and crumbs. Never use low quality steel items scraping food residue from the surface of the grill.

A grill brush with stainless steel handle would be a good investment for keeping your electric grill clean. You may also use a moist sponge and mild soap to remove tough stains.

Use a paper towel or soft kitchen cloth to dry the electric grill after cleaning to avoid electric shock.

Once the machine and all the detachable parts dry out completely, you may apply a bit of oil on the grill to keep it in prime condition.

Keep the lid tightly closed when the appliance is not in use to avoid minute particles like dust to accumulate in the pan. The grease may also attract bugs.

To make future cleanup easier, use a sheet of parchment paper or aluminum tin foil for items with heavy coatings. Make sure the food is heavy enough to weigh down the sheet as it may fly around due to the hot circulating air.

APPETIZERS AND SIDE DISHES

1.   Baked Eggplant Pepper & Mushrooms

Servings: 4
Cooking Time: 20 Minutes
Ingredients:

- 2 eggplants
- 2 cups mushrooms
- 1/4 tsp black pepper
- 4 bell peppers
- 2 tbsp olive oil
- 1 tsp salt

Directions:

1. Fit the Cuisinart oven with the rack in position
2. Cut all vegetables into the small bite-sized pieces and place in a baking dish.
3. Drizzle vegetables with olive oil and season with pepper and salt.
4. Set to bake at 390 F for 25 minutes. After 5 minutes place the baking dish in the preheated oven.
5. Serve and enjoy.
- **Nutrition Info:** Calories 87 Fat 4 g Carbohydrates 13.2 g Sugar 7.4 g Protein 2.5 g Cholesterol 0 mg

2.   Baked Asparagus

Servings: 4
Cooking Time: 15 Minutes
Ingredients:

- 30 asparagus spears, cut the ends
- 1/2 tsp garlic powder
- 1 tbsp olive oil
- Pepper
- Salt

Directions:

1. Fit the Cuisinart oven with the rack in position
2. Add asparagus into the large bowl. Drizzle with oil.
3. Sprinkle with garlic powder, pepper, and salt. Toss well.
4. Arrange asparagus in baking pan.
5. Set to bake at 400 F for 20 minutes. After 5 minutes place the baking pan in the preheated oven.
6. Serve and enjoy.

- **Nutrition Info:** Calories 67 Fat 3.7 g Carbohydrates 7.3 g Sugar 3.5 g Protein 4 g Cholesterol 0 mg

3.   Mini Salmon & Cheese Quiches

Servings:15
Cooking Time: 20 Minutes
Ingredients:

- 15 mini tart cases
- 4 eggs, lightly beaten
- ½ cup heavy cream
- Salt and black pepper
- 3 oz smoked salmon
- 6 oz cream cheese, divided into 15 pieces
- 6 fresh dill

Directions:

1. Mix together eggs and heavy cream in a pourable measuring container. Arrange the tarts on the basket. Fill them with the mixture, halfway up the side and top with salmon and cream cheese. Bake for 10 minutes at 340 F on Bake function, regularly checking to avoid overcooking. Sprinkle with dill and serve chilled.

4.   Spinach And Artichokes Sauté

Servings: 4
Cooking Time: 20 Minutes
Ingredients:

- 10 oz. artichoke hearts; halved
- 2 cups baby spinach
- 3 garlic cloves
- ¼ cup veggie stock
- 2 tsp. lime juice
- Salt and black pepper to taste.

Directions:

1. In a pan that fits your air fryer, mix all the ingredients, toss, introduce in the fryer and cook at 370°F for 15 minutes
2. Divide between plates and serve as a side dish.
- **Nutrition Info:** Calories: 209; Fat: 6g; Fiber: 2g; Carbs: 4g; Protein: 8g

5.   Green Mango Salad

Servings: 6
Cooking Time: 10 Minutes

Ingredients:

- 1/3 cup chopped cashews
- 2 mangos
- 1/3 cup chopped fresh coriander
- 1/3 cup chopped mint
- 2 tablespoons lime juice
- 4 teaspoons sugar
- 4 teaspoons fish sauce
- 1 tablespoon olive oil
- 1/4 teaspoon Asian chili sauce
- 1/4 teaspoon hot pepper sauce
- 1 sweet red pepper, thinly sliced
- 1 cup thinly sliced red onion

Directions:

1. Start by toasting cashews in toaster oven for 8 minutes.
2. Cut pointed ends off mangos, then skin.
3. Cut the mangos lengthwise into thin slices, then stack them on top of each other and cut again into thin strips.
4. In a large bowl, combine mint, coriander, lime juice, fish sauce, sugar, olive oil, and chili sauce.
5. Add mangos, red pepper, and onions to the bowl and toss.
6. Transfer salad to plates and sprinkle with cashews before serving.
- **Nutrition Info:** Calories: 140, Sodium: 317 mg, Dietary Fiber: 2.7 g, Total Fat: 6.2 g, Total Carbs: 20.7 g, Protein: 2.3 g.

6. Cheddar Cheese Cauliflower Casserole

Servings: 8
Cooking Time: 35 Minutes
Ingredients:

- 4 cups cauliflower florets
- 1 1/2 cups cheddar cheese, shredded
- 1 cup sour cream
- 4 bacon slices, cooked and crumbled
- 3 green onions, chopped

Directions:

1. Fit the Cuisinart oven with the rack in position
2. Boil water in a large pot. Add cauliflower in boiling water and cook for 8-10 minutes or until tender. Drain well.
3. Transfer cauliflower in a large bowl.

4. Add half bacon, half green onion, 1 cup cheese, and sour cream in cauliflower bowl and mix well.
5. Transfer mixture into a greased baking dish and sprinkle with remaining cheese.
6. Set to bake at 350 F for 30 minutes. After 5 minutes place the baking dish in the preheated oven.
7. Garnish with remaining green onion and bacon.
8. Serve and enjoy.
- **Nutrition Info:** Calories 213 Fat 17.1 g Carbohydrates 4.7 g Sugar 1.5 g Protein 10.8 g Cholesterol 45 mg

7. Green Beans

Servings: 4
Cooking Time: 20 Minutes
Ingredients:

- 6 cups green beans; trimmed
- 1 tbsp. hot paprika
- 2 tbsp. olive oil
- A pinch of salt and black pepper

Directions:

1. Take a bowl and mix the green beans with the other ingredients, toss, put them in the air fryer's basket and cook at 370°F for 20 minutes
2. Divide between plates and serve as a side dish.
- **Nutrition Info:** Calories: 120; Fat: 5g; Fiber: 1g; Carbs: 4g; Protein: 2g

8. Lemon-thyme Bruschetta

Servings: 10
Cooking Time: 7 Minutes
Ingredients:

- 1 baguette
- 8 ounces ricotta cheese
- 1 lemon
- Salt
- Freshly cracked black pepper
- Honey
- 8 sprigs fresh thyme

Directions:

1. Start by preheating toaster oven to 425°F.
2. Thinly slice baguette, and zest lemon.

3. Mix ricotta and lemon zest together and season with salt and pepper.
4. Toast the baguette slices for 7 minutes or until they start to brown.
5. Spread ricotta mix over slices.
6. Drizzle with honey and top with thyme, then serve.
- **Nutrition Info:** Calories: 60, Sodium: 71 mg, Dietary Fiber: 0.6 g, Total Fat: 2.0 g, Total Carbs: 7.6 g, Protein: 3.5 g.

9. Risotto Bites

Servings: 4
Cooking Time: 10 Minutes
Ingredients:
- 1½ cups cooked risotto
- 3 tablespoons Parmesan cheese, grated
- ½ egg, beaten
- 1½ oz. mozzarella cheese, cubed
- 1/3 cup breadcrumbs

Directions:
1. In a bowl, add the risotto, Parmesan and egg and mix until well combined.
2. Make 20 equal-sized balls from the mixture.
3. Insert a mozzarella cube in the center of each ball.
4. With your fingers smooth the risotto mixture to cover the ball.
5. In a shallow dish, place the breadcrumbs.
6. Coat the balls with the breadcrumbs evenly.
7. Press "Power Button" of Air Fry Oven and turn the dial to select the "Air Fry" mode.
8. Press the Time button and again turn the dial to set the cooking time to 10 minutes.
9. Now push the Temp button and rotate the dial to set the temperature at 390 degrees F.
10. Press "Start/Pause" button to start.
11. When the unit beeps to show that it is preheated, open the lid.
12. Arrange the balls in "Air Fry Basket" and insert in the oven.
13. Serve warm.
- **Nutrition Info:** Calories 340 Total Fat 4.3 g Saturated Fat 2 g Cholesterol 29 mg Sodium 173 mg Total Carbs 62.4 g Fiber 1.3 g Sugar 0.7 g Protein 11.3 g

10. Party Pull Apart

Servings: 10
Cooking Time: 20 Minutes
Ingredients:
- 5 cloves garlic
- 1/3 cup fresh parsley
- 2 tbsp. olive oil
- 4 oz. mozzarella cheese, sliced
- 3 tbsp. butter
- 1/8 tsp salt
- 1 loaf sour dough bread

Directions:
1. Place the rack in position 1 of the oven.
2. In a food processor, add garlic, parsley, and oil and pulse until garlic is chopped fine.
3. Stack the mozzarella cheese and cut into 1-inch squares.
4. Heat the butter in a small saucepan over medium heat. Add the garlic mixture and salt and cook 2 minutes, stirring occasionally. Remove from heat.
5. Use a sharp, serrated knife to make 1-inch diagonal cuts across the bread being careful not to cut all the way through.
6. With a spoon, drizzle garlic butter into the cuts in the bread. Stack 3-4 cheese squares and place in each of the cuts.
7. Place the bread on a sheet of foil and fold up the sides. Cut a second piece of foil just big enough to cover the top.
8. Set oven to convection bake on 350°F for 25 minutes. After 5 minutes, place the bread in the oven and bake 10 minutes.
9. Remove the top piece of foil and bake 10 minutes more until the cheese has completely melted. Serve immediately.
- **Nutrition Info:** Calories 173, Total Fat 7g, Saturated Fat 3g, Total Carbs 18g, Net Carbs 17g, Protein 7g, Sugar 2g, Fiber 1g, Sodium 337mg, Potassium 68mg, Phosphorus 112mg

11. Rosemary Potato Chips

Servings:4
Cooking Time: 30 Minutes
Ingredients:
- 1 pound potatoes, cut into thin slices
- ¼ cup olive oil

- 1 tbsp garlic puree
- ½ cup heavy cream
- 2 tbsp fresh rosemary, chopped

Directions:

1. Preheat Breville on AirFry function to 390 F. In a bowl, mix oil, garlic puree, and salt. Add in the potato slices and toss to coat. Lay the potato slices onto the frying basket and place in the oven. Press Start and cook for 20-25 minutes. Sprinkle with rosemary and serve.

12. Air Fried Green Tomatoes(1)

Servings: 4
Cooking Time: 20 Minutes
Ingredients:

- 2 medium green tomatoes
- ⅓ cup grated Parmesan cheese.
- ¼ cup blanched finely ground almond flour.
- 1 large egg.

Directions:

1. Slice tomatoes into ½-inch-thick slices. Take a medium bowl, whisk the egg. Take a large bowl, mix the almond flour and Parmesan.
2. Dip each tomato slice into the egg, then dredge in the almond flour mixture. Place the slices into the air fryer basket
3. Adjust the temperature to 400 Degrees F and set the timer for 7 minutes. Flip the slices halfway through the cooking time. Serve immediately
- **Nutrition Info:** Calories: 106; Protein: 6.2g; Fiber: 1.4g; Fat: 6.7g; Carbs: 5.9g

13. Tasty Hassel Back Potatoes

Servings: 4
Cooking Time: 30 Minutes
Ingredients:

- 4 potatoes, peel & cut potato across the potato to make 1/8-inch slices
- 1/4 cup parmesan cheese, shredded
- 1 tbsp olive oil

Directions:

1. Fit the Cuisinart oven with the rack in position 2.
2. Brush potatoes with olive oil.

3. Place potatoes in the air fryer basket then place an air fryer basket in the baking pan.
4. Place a baking pan on the oven rack. Set to air fry at 350 F for 30 minutes.
5. Sprinkle cheese on top of potatoes and serve.
- **Nutrition Info:** Calories 195 Fat 4.9 g Carbohydrates 33.7 g Sugar 2.5 g Protein 5.4 g Cholesterol 4 mg

14. Salty Baked Almonds

Servings: 4
Cooking Time: 25 Minutes
Ingredients:

- 1 cup raw almonds
- 1 egg white, beaten
- ½ teaspoon coarse sea salt

Directions:

1. Spread the almonds in the baking pan in an even layer.
2. Slide the baking pan into Rack Position 1, select Convection Bake, set temperature to 350ºF (180ºC) and set time to 20 minutes.
3. When cooking is complete, the almonds should be lightly browned and fragrant. Remove from the oven.
4. Coat the almonds with the egg white and sprinkle with the salt. Return the pan to the oven.
5. Slide the baking pan into Rack Position 1, select Convection Bake, set temperature to 350ºF (180ºC) and set time to 5 minutes.
6. When cooking is complete, the almonds should be dried. Cool completely before serving.

15. Sausage Mushroom Caps(2)

Servings: 2
Cooking Time: 20 Minutes
Ingredients:

- ½ lb. Italian sausage
- 6 large Portobello mushroom caps
- ¼ cup grated Parmesan cheese.
- ¼ cup chopped onion
- 2 tbsp. blanched finely ground almond flour
- 1 tsp. minced fresh garlic

Directions:

1. Use a spoon to hollow out each mushroom cap, reserving scrapings.
2. In a medium skillet over medium heat, brown the sausage about 10 minutes or until fully cooked and no pink remains. Drain and then add reserved mushroom scrapings, onion, almond flour, Parmesan and garlic.
3. Gently fold ingredients together and continue cooking an additional minute, then remove from heat
4. Evenly spoon the mixture into mushroom caps and place the caps into a 6-inch round pan. Place pan into the air fryer basket
5. Adjust the temperature to 375 Degrees F and set the timer for 8 minutes. When finished cooking, the tops will be browned and bubbling. Serve warm.
- **Nutrition Info:** Calories: 404; Protein: 24.3g; Fiber: 4.5g; Fat: 25.8g; Carbs: 18.2g

16. Stuffed Mushrooms With Rice & Cheese

Servings: 10
Cooking Time: 30 Minutes
Ingredients:
- 10 Swiss brown mushrooms
- 2 tbsp olive oil
- 1 cup cooked brown rice
- 1 cup grated Grana Padano cheese
- 1 tsp dried mixed herbs
- Salt and black pepper to taste

Directions:
1. Brush mushrooms with oil and arrange onto the Cuisinart Air Fryer baking tray. In a bowl, mix rice, Grana Padano cheese, herbs, salt, and pepper. Stuff the mushrooms with the mixture. Cook in the oven for 14 minutes at 360 F on Bake function until the cheese has melted. Serve.

17. Avocado Fries

Servings: 4
Cooking Time: 20 Minutes
Ingredients:
- 1 oz. pork rinds, finely ground
- 2 medium avocados

Directions:

1. Cut each avocado in half. Remove the pit. Carefully remove the peel and then slice the flesh into ¼-inch-thick slices.
2. Place the pork rinds into a medium bowl and press each piece of avocado into the pork rinds to coat completely. Place the avocado pieces into the air fryer basket. Adjust the temperature to 350 Degrees F and set the timer for 5 minutes. Serve immediately
- **Nutrition Info:** Calories: 153; Protein: 4g; Fiber: 6g; Fat: 19g; Carbs: 9g

18. Crusted Brussels Sprouts With Sage

Servings:4
Cooking Time: 15 Minutes
Ingredients:
- 1 pound (454 g) Brussels sprouts, halved
- 1 cup bread crumbs
- 2 tablespoons grated Grana Padano cheese
- 1 tablespoon paprika
- 2 tablespoons canola oil
- 1 tablespoon chopped sage

Directions:
1. Line the air fryer basket with parchment paper. Set aside.
2. In a small bowl, thoroughly mix the bread crumbs, cheese, and paprika. In a large bowl, place the Brussels sprouts and drizzle the canola oil over the top. Sprinkle with the bread crumb mixture and toss to coat.
3. Transfer the Brussels sprouts to the prepared basket.
4. Put the air fryer basket on the baking pan and slide into Rack Position 2, select Roast, set temperature to 400ºF (205ºC), and set time to 15 minutes.
5. Stir the Brussels a few times during cooking.
6. When cooking is complete, the Brussels sprouts should be lightly browned and crisp. Transfer the Brussels sprouts to a plate and sprinkle the sage on top before serving.

19. Baked Vegetables

Servings: 6
Cooking Time: 30 Minutes
Ingredients:
- 2 zucchini, sliced

- 2 tomatoes, quartered
- 6 fresh basil leaves, sliced
- 2 tsp Italian seasoning
- 2 tbsp olive oil
- 1 eggplant, sliced
- 1 onion, sliced
- 1 bell pepper, cut into strips
- Pepper
- Salt

Directions:
1. Fit the Cuisinart oven with the rack in position
2. Add all ingredients except basil leaves into the bowl and toss well.
3. Transfer vegetable mixture in parchment-lined baking pan.
4. Set to bake at 400 F for 35 minutes. After 5 minutes place the baking pan in the preheated oven.
5. Garnish with basil and serve.
- **Nutrition Info:** Calories 96 Fat 5.5 g Carbohydrates 11.7 g Sugar 6.4 g Protein 2.3 g Cholesterol 1 mg

20. Baked Honey Carrots

Servings: 4
Cooking Time: 25 Minutes
Ingredients:
- 1 lb baby carrots
- 2 tbsp butter, melted
- 3 tbsp honey
- 2 tsp fresh parsley, chopped
- 1 tbsp Dijon mustard
- Pepper
- Salt

Directions:
1. Fit the Cuisinart oven with the rack in position
2. In a large bowl, toss carrots with Dijon mustard, honey, butter, pepper, and salt.
3. Transfer carrots in a baking dish and spread evenly.
4. Set to bake at 400 F for 30 minutes. After 5 minutes place the baking dish in the preheated oven.
5. Serve and enjoy.

- **Nutrition Info:** Calories 141 Fat 6.1 g Carbohydrates 22.6 g Sugar 18.4 g Protein 1 g Cholesterol 15 mg

21. Butternut And Apple Mash

Servings: 4
Cooking Time: 15 Minutes
Ingredients:
- 1 butternut squash, peeled and cut into medium chunks
- 2 apples, cored and sliced
- 1 cup water
- ½ teaspoon apple pie spice
- Salt, to taste
- 2 tablespoons butter, browned
- 1 yellow onion, thinly sliced

Directions:
1. Place the pieces of pumpkin, onion and apple in the steam basket of the Instant Pot, add the water to the Instant Pot, cover and cook for 8 minutes in manual setting.
2. Quickly release the pressure and transfer the pumpkin, onion and apple to a bowl. Smash everything with a potato masher, add salt, apple pie spices and brown butter, mix well and serve hot.
- **Nutrition Info:** Calories: 140, Fat: 2.3, Fiber: 6.5, Carbohydrate: 24, Proteins: 2.5

22. Mustard Chicken Wings

Servings:4
Cooking Time: 30 Minutes
Ingredients:
- ½ tsp celery salt
- ½ tsp bay leaf powder
- ½ tsp ground black pepper
- ½ tsp paprika
- ¼ tsp dry mustard
- ¼ tsp cayenne pepper
- ¼ tsp allspice
- 2 pounds chicken wings

Directions:
1. Preheat Breville to 400 F on AirFry function. In a bowl, mix celery salt, bay leaf powder, black pepper, paprika, dry mustard, cayenne pepper, and allspice. Add in the wings and toss to coat.

2. Arrange the wings in an even layer on the basket. Press Start and AirFry the chicken until it's no longer pink around the bone, about 20-25 minutes until crispy on the outside. Serve.

23. Butterbeans With Feta & Bacon

Servings:2
Cooking Time: 20 Minutes
Ingredients:
- 1 (14 oz) can butter beans
- 1 tbsp fresh chives, chopped
- ½ cup feta cheese, crumbled
- Black pepper to taste
- 1 tsp olive oil
- 2 oz bacon, sliced

Directions:
1. Preheat Breville on AirFry function to 340 F. Blitz beans, oil, and pepper in a small blender. Arrange bacon slices on the frying basket.
2. Top with chives and place in the oven. Press Start and cook for 12 minutes. Add feta to the bean mixture and stir. Serve bacon with the dip.

24. Baked Cauliflower & Tomatoes

Servings: 4
Cooking Time: 20 Minutes
Ingredients:
- 4 cups cauliflower florets
- 1 tbsp capers, drained
- 3 tbsp olive oil
- 1/2 cup cherry tomatoes, halved
- 2 tbsp fresh parsley, chopped
- 2 garlic cloves, sliced
- Pepper
- Salt

Directions:
1. Fit the Cuisinart oven with the rack in position
2. In a bowl, toss together cherry tomatoes, cauliflower, oil, garlic, capers, pepper, and salt and spread in baking pan.
3. Set to bake at 450 F for 25 minutes. After 5 minutes place the baking pan in the preheated oven.
4. Garnish with parsley and serve.

- **Nutrition Info:** Calories 123 Fat 10.7 g Carbohydrates 6.9 g Sugar 3 g Protein 2.4 g Cholesterol 0 mg

25. Asparagus Wrapped In Bacon

Servings:4
Cooking Time: 25 Minutes
Ingredients:
- 20 spears asparagus
- 4 bacon slices
- 1 tbsp olive oil
- 1 tbsp sesame oil
- 1 garlic clove, minced

Directions:
1. Preheat Breville on AirFry function to 380 F. In a bowl, mix the oils, sugar, and garlic. Separate the asparagus into 4 bunches (5 spears in 1 bunch) and wrap each bunch with a bacon slice.
2. Drizzle the bunches with oil mix. Put them in the frying basket and place in the oven. Press Start and cook for 8 minutes. Serve warm.

26. Three Bean Medley

Servings: 4
Cooking Time: 15 Minutes
Ingredients:
- 4 cups water
- 1 cup garbanzo beans, soaked overnight and drained
- 1 cup cranberry beans, soaked overnight and drained
- 1½ cups green beans
- 1 garlic clove, peeled and crushed
- 1 bay leaf
- 1 small red onion, peeled and chopped
- 1 tablespoon sugar
- 2 celery stalks, chopped
- 1 bunch parsley, chopped
- Salt and ground black pepper, to taste
- 5 tablespoons apple cider vinegar
- 4 tablespoons extra virgin olive oil

Directions:
1. Place the water in the Instant Pot. Add the bay leaf, garlic and chickpeas. Also place the basket in the pan and add the cranberries.

2. Wrap the green beans in aluminum foil and place them in the steam basket. Cover the Instant Pot and cook in the Bean / Chili setting for 15 minutes.
3. Release the pressure naturally for 10 minutes, uncover the Instant Pot, drain the beans, discard them and place them all in a bowl. In another bowl, mix the onion with the vinegar and sugar, mix well and set aside for a few minutes.
4. Add the onion to the beans and mix well. Also add celery, olive oil, salt, pepper to taste and parsley, mix well, divide between plates and serve.
- **Nutrition Info:** Calories: 200, Fat: 1, Fiber: 6, Carbohydrate: 45, Proteins: 4

27. Lemon-garlic Kale Salad

Servings: 8
Cooking Time: 10 Minutes
Ingredients:
- 2 cups sliced almonds
- 1/3 cup lemon juice
- 1 teaspoon salt
- 1-1/2 cups olive oil
- 4 cloves crushed garlic
- 12 ounces kale, stems removed

Directions:
1. Set toaster oven to toast and toast almonds for about 5 minutes.
2. Combine lemon juice and salt in a small bowl, then add olive oil and garlic; mix well and set aside.
3. Slice kale into thin ribbons; place in a bowl and sprinkle with almonds.
4. Remove garlic from dressing, then add desired amount of dressing to kale and toss.
5. Add additional dressing if necessary, and serve.
- **Nutrition Info:** Calories: 487, Sodium: 312 mg, Dietary Fiber: 3.7 g, Total Fat: 49.8 g, Total Carbs: 10.2 g, Protein: 6.5 g.

28. Potato Chips With Lemony Dip

Servings: 3
Cooking Time: 25 Minutes
Ingredients:
- 3 large potatoes, sliced

- 1 cup sour cream
- 2 scallions, white part minced
- 3 tbsp olive oil.
- ½ tsp lemon juice
- salt and black pepper

Directions:
1. Preheat Cuisinart on Air Fry function to 350 F. Place the potatoes into the AirFryer basket Cuisinart and fit in the baking tray. Cook for 15 minutes, flipping once. Season with salt and pepper. Mix sour cream, olive oil, scallions, lemon juice, salt, and pepper and serve with chips.

29. Baked Italian Vegetables

Servings: 6
Cooking Time: 30 Minutes
Ingredients:
- 1 eggplant, sliced
- 1 onion, sliced
- 1 potato, peel & cut into chunks
- 1 bell pepper, cut into strips
- 2 zucchini, sliced
- 2 tomatoes, quartered
- 5 fresh basil leaves, sliced
- 2 tsp Italian seasoning
- 2 tbsp olive oil
- Pepper
- Salt

Directions:
1. Fit the Cuisinart oven with the rack in position
2. Add all ingredients except basil leaves into the mixing bowl and toss well.
3. Transfer vegetable mixture on a prepared baking pan.
4. Set to bake at 400 F for 35 minutes. After 5 minutes place the baking dish in the preheated oven.
5. Garnish with basil leaves and serve.
- **Nutrition Info:** Calories 117 Fat 5.6 g Carbohydrates 16.6 g Sugar 6.6 g Protein 2.9 g Cholesterol 1 mg

30. Baked Artichoke Hearts

Servings: 6
Cooking Time: 25 Minutes
Ingredients:

- 15 oz frozen artichoke hearts, defrosted
- 1 tbsp olive oil
- Pepper
- Salt

Directions:
1. Fit the Cuisinart oven with the rack in position
2. Arrange artichoke hearts in baking pan and drizzle with olive oil. Season with pepper and salt.
3. Set to bake at 400 F for 30 minutes. After 5 minutes place the baking pan in the preheated oven.
4. Serve and enjoy.
- **Nutrition Info:** Calories 53 Fat 2.4 g Carbohydrates 7.5 g Sugar 0.7 g Protein 2.3 g Cholesterol 0 mg

31. Baked Ratatouille

Servings: 6
Cooking Time: 55 Minutes
Ingredients:
- 1 large eggplant, steamed and sliced
- 1/4 tsp dried thyme
- 2 bell pepper, sliced
- 4 tomatoes, sliced
- 2 tbsp olive oil
- 4 medium zucchini, sliced
- 1 tsp dried basil
- 1/2 tsp dried oregano

Directions:
1. Fit the Cuisinart oven with the rack in position
2. Add all vegetable slices to a large bowl and season with salt and drizzle with oil.
3. Layer vegetable slices into the greased baking dish.
4. Set to bake at 400 F for 60 minutes. After 5 minutes place the baking dish in the preheated oven.
5. Sprinkle with dried herbs.
6. Serve and enjoy.
- **Nutrition Info:** Calories 108 Fat 5.3 g Carbohydrates 15.2 g Sugar 8.7 g Protein 3.5 g Cholesterol 0 mg

32. Savory Parsley Crab Cakes

Servings: 6

Cooking Time: 20 Minutes
Ingredients:
- 1 lb crab meat, shredded
- 2 eggs, beaten
- ½ cup breadcrumbs
- ⅓ cup finely chopped green onion
- ¼ cup parsley, chopped
- 1 tbsp mayonnaise
- 1 tsp sweet chili sauce
- ½ tsp paprika
- Salt and black pepper to taste

Directions:
1. In a bowl, add crab meat, eggs, crumbs, green onion, parsley, mayo, chili sauce, paprika, salt and black pepper; mix well with your hands.
2. Shape into 6 cakes and grease them lightly with oil. Arrange them in the fryer basket without overcrowding. Fit in the baking tray and cook for 8 minutes at 400 F on Air Fry function, turning once halfway through.

33. Sunday Calamari Rings

Servings:4
Cooking Time: 20 Minutes
Ingredients:
- 1 lb calamari (squid), cut in rings
- ¼ cup flour
- 2 large beaten eggs
- 1 cup breadcrumbs

Directions:
1. Coat the calamari rings with the flour and dip them in the eggs. Then, roll in the breadcrumbs. Refrigerate for 2 hours. Line them in the frying basket and spray with cooking spray.
2. Select AirFry function, adjust the temperature to 380 F, and press Start. Cook for 14 minutes. Serve with garlic mayo and lemon wedges.

34. Parmesan Cabbage Wedges

Servings:4
Cooking Time: 30 Minutes
Ingredients:
- ½ head cabbage, cut into wedges
- 4 tbsp butter, melted
- 2 cup Parmesan cheese, grated

- Salt and black pepper to taste
- 1 tsp smoked paprika

Directions:

1. Preheat Breville on AirFry function to 330 F. Line a baking sheet with parchment paper. Brush the cabbage wedges with butter and season with salt and pepper.
2. Coat the cabbage with the Parmesan cheese and arrange on the baking sheet; sprinkle with paprika. Press Start and cook for 15 minutes. Flip the wedges over and cook for an additional 10 minutes. Serve with yogurt dip.

35. Scallion & Cheese Sandwich

Servings:1
Cooking Time: 15 Minutes
Ingredients:

- 2 tbsp Parmesan cheese, shredded
- 1 tsp fresh scallions, chopped
- 1 tbsp butter
- 2 slices bread
- ¾ cup cheddar cheese

Directions:

1. Preheat Breville on AirFry function to 360 F. Lay the bread slices on a flat surface. Spread the exposed side with butter, followed by some cheddar cheese, and scallions. On the other slice, spread butter and then sprinkle the remaining cheddar cheese.
2. Bring the buttered sides together to form sandwich. Place the sandwich in baking tray and place in the oven. Press Start and cook for 10 minutes. Serve with berry sauce.

36. Polenta Sticks

Servings: 4
Cooking Time: 6 Minutes
Ingredients:

- 1 tablespoon oil
- 2½ cups cooked polenta
- Salt, to taste
- ¼ cup Parmesan cheese

Directions:

1. Place the polenta in a lightly greased baking pan.
2. With a plastic wrap, cover and refrigerate for about 1 hour or until set.

3. Remove from the refrigerator and cut into desired sized slices.
4. Sprinkle with salt.
5. Press "Power Button" of Air Fry Oven and turn the dial to select the "Air Fry" mode.
6. Press the Time button and again turn the dial to set the cooking time to 6 minutes.
7. Now push the Temp button and rotate the dial to set the temperature at 350 degrees F.
8. Press "Start/Pause" button to start.
9. When the unit beeps to show that it is preheated, open the lid.
10. Arrange the pan over the "Wire Rack" and insert in the oven.
11. Top with cheese and serve.

- **Nutrition Info:** Calories 397 Total Fat 5.6g Saturated Fat 1.3 g Cholesterol 4mg Sodium 127 mg Total Carbs 76.2 g Fiber 2.5 g Sugar 1 g Protein 9.1 g

37. Sausage Mushroom Caps(3)

Servings: 2
Cooking Time: 8 Minutes
Ingredients:

- ½ lb. Italian sausage
- 6 large Portobello mushroom caps
- ¼ cup grated Parmesan cheese.
- ¼ cup chopped onion
- 2 tbsp. blanched finely ground almond flour
- 1 tsp. minced fresh garlic

Directions:

1. Use a spoon to hollow out each mushroom cap, reserving scrapings.
2. In a medium skillet over medium heat, brown the sausage about 10 minutes or until fully cooked and no pink remains. Drain and then add reserved mushroom scrapings, onion, almond flour, Parmesan and garlic.
3. Gently fold ingredients together and continue cooking an additional minute, then remove from heat
4. Evenly spoon the mixture into mushroom caps and place the caps into a 6-inch round pan. Place pan into the air fryer basket
5. Adjust the temperature to 375 Degrees F and set the timer for 8 minutes. When

finished cooking, the tops will be browned and bubbling. Serve warm.

- **Nutrition Info:** Calories: 404; Protein: 24.3g; Fiber: 4.5g; Fat: 25.8g; Carbs: 18.2g

38. Healthy Spinach Muffins

Servings: 12
Cooking Time: 15 Minutes
Ingredients:

- 10 eggs
- 2 cups spinach, chopped
- 1/2 tsp dried basil
- 1 1/2 cups parmesan cheese, grated
- 1/4 tsp garlic powder
- 1/4 tsp onion powder
- Salt

Directions:

1. Fit the Cuisinart oven with the rack in position
2. Spray 12-cups muffin tin with cooking spray and set aside.
3. In a large bowl, whisk eggs with basil, garlic powder, onion powder, and salt.
4. Add cheese and spinach and stir well.
5. Pour egg mixture into the prepared muffin tin.
6. Set to bake at 400 F for 20 minutes. After 5 minutes place muffin tin in the preheated oven.
7. Serve and enjoy.

- **Nutrition Info:** Calories 90 Fat 6.1 g Carbohydrates 0.9 g Sugar 0.3 g Protein 8.4 g Cholesterol 144 mg

39. French Fries

Servings: 4
Cooking Time: 10 Minutes
Ingredients:

- ¼ teaspoon baking soda Oil for frying
- Salt, to taste
- 8 medium potatoes, peeled, cut into medium matchsticks, and patted dry
- 1 cup water

Directions:

1. Put the water in the Instant Pot, add the salt and baking soda and mix. Place the potatoes in the steam basket and place them in the Instant Pot, cover and cook with manual adjustment for 3 minutes.
2. Release the pressure naturally, remove the chips from the Instant Pot and place them in a bowl. Heat a pan with enough oil over medium-high heat, add the potatoes, spread and cook until they are golden brown.
3. Transfer the potatoes to the paper towels to drain the excess fat and place them in a bowl. Salt, mix well and serve.

- **Nutrition Info:** Calories: 300, Fat: 10, Fiber: 3.7, Carbohydrate: 41, Proteins: 3.4

BREAKFAST RECIPES

40. Healthy Oatmeal Bars

Servings: 18
Cooking Time: 20 Minutes
Ingredients:

- 2 cups oatmeal
- 1/2 tsp allspice
- 1 tsp baking soda
- 1 tbsp maple syrup
- 1 cup butter
- 1 cup of sugar
- 1 cup flour

Directions:

1. Fit the Cuisinart oven with the rack in position
2. Add butter and maple syrup into a bowl and microwave until butter is melted. Stir well.
3. In a mixing bowl, mix oatmeal, sugar, flour, allspice, and baking soda.
4. Add melted butter and maple syrup mixture and mix until well combined.
5. Pour mixture into the parchment-lined 9*12-inch baking dish. Spread well.
6. Set to bake at 350 F for 25 minutes, after 5 minutes, place the baking dish in the oven.
7. Slice and serve.
- **Nutrition Info:** Calories 195 Fat 10.9 g Carbohydrates 23.4 g Sugar 11.9 g Protein 2 g Cholesterol 27 mg

41. Caprese Sourdough Sandwich

Servings: 2
Cooking Time: 25 Minutes
Ingredients:

- 4 sourdough bread slices
- 2 tbsp mayonnaise
- 2 slices ham
- 2 lettuce leaves
- 1 tomato, sliced
- 2 mozzarella cheese slices
- Salt and black pepper to taste

Directions:

1. On a clean board, lay the sourdough slices and spread with mayonnaise. Top 2 of the slices with ham, lettuce, tomato and mozzarella. Season with salt and pepper. Top with the remaining two slices to form

two sandwiches. Spray with oil and transfer to the frying basket. Cook in the preheated Breville oven for 14 minutes at 340 F on Bake function.

42. Prawn And Cabbage Egg Rolls Wraps

Servings: 4
Cooking Time: 18 Minutes
Ingredients:

- 2 tablespoons olive oil
- 1 carrot, cut into strips
- 1-inch piece fresh ginger, grated
- 1 tablespoon minced garlic
- 2 tablespoons soy sauce
- ¼ cup chicken broth
- 1 tablespoon sugar
- 1 cup shredded Napa cabbage
- 1 tablespoon sesame oil
- 8 cooked prawns, minced
- 8 egg roll wrappers
- 1 egg, beaten
- Cooking spray

Directions:

1. Spritz the air fryer basket with cooking spray. Set aside.
2. Heat the olive oil in a nonstick skillet over medium heat until shimmering.
3. Add the carrot, ginger, and garlic and sauté for 2 minutes or until fragrant.
4. Pour in the soy sauce, broth, and sugar. Bring to a boil. Keep stirring.
5. Add the cabbage and simmer for 4 minutes or until the cabbage is tender.
6. Turn off the heat and mix in the sesame oil. Let sit for 15 minutes.
7. Use a strainer to remove the vegetables from the liquid, then combine with the minced prawns.
8. Unfold the egg roll wrappers on a clean work surface, then divide the prawn mixture in the center of wrappers.
9. Dab the edges of a wrapper with the beaten egg, then fold a corner over the filling and tuck the corner under the filling. Fold the left and right corner into the center. Roll the wrapper up and press to seal. Repeat with remaining wrappers.

10. Arrange the wrappers in the pan and spritz with cooking spray.
11. Put the air fryer basket on the baking pan and slide into Rack Position 2, select Air Fry, set temperature to 370ºF (188ºC) and set time to 12 minutes.
12. Flip the wrappers halfway through the cooking time.
13. When cooking is complete, the wrappers should be golden.
14. Serve immediately.

43. Vanilla & Cinnamon Toast Toppet

Servings: 6
Cooking Time: 10 Minutes
Ingredients:
- 12 slices bread
- ½ cup sugar
- 1 ½ tsp cinnamon
- 1 stick of butter, softened
- 1 tsp vanilla extract

Directions:
1. Preheat Cuisinart on Toast function to 360 F. Combine all ingredients, except the bread, in a bowl. Spread the buttery cinnamon mixture onto the bread slices. Place the bread slices in the toaster oven. Cook for 8 minutes. Serve.

44. Raspberries Maple Pancakes

Servings: 4
Cooking Time: 15 Minutes
Ingredients:
- 2 cups all-purpose flour
- 1 cup milk
- 3 eggs, beaten
- 1 tsp baking powder
- 1 cup brown sugar
- 1 ½ tsp vanilla extract
- ½ cup frozen raspberries, thawed
- 2 tbsp maple syrup
- A pinch of salt

Directions:
1. Preheat Cuisinart on Bake function to 400 F. In a bowl, mix the flour, baking powder, salt, milk, eggs, vanilla extract, and sugar until smooth. Stir in the raspberries. Do it gently to avoid coloring the batter.

2. Grease a pie pan with cooking spray. Drop the batter onto the pan. Make sure to leave some space between the pancakes. Cook for 10-15 minutes. Drizzle with maple syrup and serve.

45. Spicy Egg Casserole

Servings: 8
Cooking Time: 45 Minutes
Ingredients:
- 10 eggs
- 1 cup Colby jack cheese, shredded
- 1 cup cottage cheese
- 1 tsp baking powder
- 1/3 cup flour
- 1/2 cup milk
- 4.5 oz can green chilies, chopped
- 1/2 small onion, minced
- 2 tbsp butter
- 1 tsp seasoned salt

Directions:
1. Fit the Cuisinart oven with the rack in position
2. Spray 9*13-inch casserole dish with cooking spray and set aside.
3. Melt butter in a pan over medium heat.
4. Add onion and green chilies and sauté for 5 minutes. Remove pan from heat and set aside.
5. In a small bowl, whisk milk, baking powder, and flour until smooth.
6. In a mixing bowl, whisk eggs with cheese, cottage cheese, and seasoned salt.
7. Add sautéed onion and green chilies, milk, and flour mixture to the eggs and whisk until well combined.
8. Pour egg mixture into the prepared casserole dish.
9. Set to bake at 350 F for 50 minutes. After 5 minutes place the casserole dish in the preheated oven.
10. Serve and enjoy.
- **Nutrition Info:** Calories 219 Fat 13.8 g Carbohydrates 8.4 g Sugar 1.4 g Protein 14.9 g Cholesterol 228 mg

46. Cinnamon French Toasts

Servings: 2

Cooking Time: 5 Minutes
Ingredients:
- 2 eggs
- ¼ cup whole milk
- 3 tablespoons sugar
- 2 teaspoons olive oil
- 1/8 teaspoon vanilla extract
- 1/8 teaspoon ground cinnamon
- 4 bread slices

Directions:
1. In a large bowl, mix together all the ingredients except bread slices.
2. Coat the bread slices with egg mixture evenly.
3. Press "Power Button" of Air Fry Oven and turn the dial to select the "Air Fry" mode.
4. Press the Time button and again turn the dial to set the cooking time to 6 minutes.
5. Now push the Temp button and rotate the dial to set the temperature at 390 degrees F.
6. Press "Start/Pause" button to start.
7. When the unit beeps to show that it is preheated, open the lid and lightly, grease the sheet pan.
8. Arrange the bread slices into "Air Fry Basket" and insert in the oven.
9. Flip the bread slices once halfway through.
10. Serve warm.
- **Nutrition Info:** Calories: 238 Cal Total Fat: 10.6 g Saturated Fat: 2.7 g Cholesterol: 167 mg Sodium: 122 mg Total Carbs: 20.8 g Fiber: 0.5 g Sugar: 0.9 g Protein: 7.9 g

47. Easy Parsnip Hash Browns

Servings:2
Cooking Time: 20 Minutes
Ingredients:
- 1 large parsnip, grated
- 3 eggs, beaten
- ½ tsp garlic powder
- ¼ tsp nutmeg
- 1 tbsp olive oil
- 1 cup flour
- Salt and black pepper to taste

Directions:
1. In a bowl, combine flour, eggs, parsnip, nutmeg, and garlic powder. Season with salt and pepper. Form patties out of the mixture.

Drizzle the basket with olive oil and arrange the patties inside. Press Start. Cook for 15 minutes on AirFry function at 360 F. Serve with garlic mayo.

48. Middle Eastern Shakshuka With Smoked Paprika

Servings:x
Cooking Time:x
Ingredients:
- 2 Tbsp olive oil
- ½ yellow onion, diced
- 1 small serrano or jalapeno chili, seeds removed, diced
- 1 tsp cumin
- 1 tsp paprika
- ½ tsp smoked paprika
- ¼ tsp coriander
- 2 eggs
- 1 can chopped tomatoes
- ½ green pepper, diced
- Salt and pepper, to taste
- Chopped parsley or cilantro

Directions:
1. Preheat Breville smart oven over medium heat.
2. Heat olive oil and saute onion until softened.
3. Add tomatoes, green pepper and chili. Cook for 4-5 minutes.
4. Add seasonings and cook for several minutes until liquid slightly reduces.
5. Make two indentations in mixture and crack eggs into them. Cover and
6. cook until eggs are done.
7. Sprinkle with salt, pepper, parsley and cilantro and serve while bubbly and hot.

49. Strawberry Cheesecake Pastries

Servings: 6
Cooking Time: 20 Minutes
Ingredients:
- 1 sheet puff pastry, thawed
- ¼ cup cream cheese, soft
- 1 tbsp. strawberry jam
- 1 ½ cups strawberries, sliced
- 1 egg
- 1 tbsp. water
- 6 tsp powdered sugar, sifted

Directions:

1. Line the baking pan with parchment paper.
2. Lay the puff pastry on a cutting board and cut into 6 rectangles. Transfer to prepared pan, placing them 1-inch apart.
3. Lightly score the pastry, creating a ½-inch border, do not cut all the way through. Use a fork to prick the center.
4. In a small bowl, combine cream cheese and jam until thoroughly combined. Spoon mixture evenly into centers of the pastry and spread it within the scored area.
5. Top pastries with sliced berries.
6. In a small bowl, whisk together egg and water. Brush edges of pastry with the egg wash.
7. Set to bake at 350°F for 20 minutes. After 5 minutes, place the baking pan in position 1 and bake pastries until golden brown and puffed.
8. Remove from oven and let cool. Dust with powdered sugar before serving.
- **Nutrition Info:** Calories 205, Total Fat 13g, Saturated Fat 4g, Total Carbs 19g, Net Carbs 18g, Protein 3g, Sugar 6g, Fiber 1g, Sodium 107mg, Potassium 97mg, Phosphorus 50mg

50. Tasty Cheddar Omelet

Servings: 1
Cooking Time: 20 Minutes
Ingredients:

- 2 eggs
- 2 tbsp cheddar cheese, grated
- 1 tsp soy sauce
- ½ onion, sliced
- Salt and black pepper to taste
- 1 tbsp olive oil

Directions:

1. Preheat Cuisinart on Bake function to 350 F. Whisk the eggs with soy sauce, salt, and pepper. Stir in onion. Grease a baking dish with the olive oil and add in the egg mixture. Cook for 10-14 minutes. Top with the grated cheddar cheese and serve.

51. Chicken Breakfast Sausages

Servings: 8 Patties
Cooking Time: 10 Minutes

Ingredients:

- 1 Granny Smith apple, peeled and finely chopped
- 2 tablespoons apple juice
- 2 garlic cloves, minced
- 1 egg white
- $^1/_3$ cup minced onion
- 3 tablespoons ground almonds
- ⅛ teaspoon freshly ground black pepper
- 1 pound (454 g) ground chicken breast

Directions:

1. Combine all the ingredients except the chicken in a medium mixing bowl and stir well.
2. Add the chicken breast to the apple mixture and mix with your hands until well incorporated.
3. Divide the mixture into 8 equal portions and shape into patties. Arrange the patties in the air fryer basket.
4. Put the air fryer basket on the baking pan and slide into Rack Position 2, select Air Fry, set temperature to 330ºF (166ºC) and set time to 10 minutes.
5. When done, a meat thermometer inserted in the center of the chicken should reach at least 165ºF (74ºC).
6. Remove from the oven to a plate. Let the chicken cool for 5 minutes and serve warm.

52. Cinnamon Streusel Bread

Servings: 8
Cooking Time: 30 Minutes
Ingredients:

- 1 cup warm water
- 1 envelope yeast, quick rising
- 1/3 cup + 6 tsp milk, divided
- 1 egg
- 3 tbsp. sugar
- 3 ½ cups flour, divided
- 1 tbsp. + 2 tsp olive oil
- 1 tsp salt
- 2 tbsp. cinnamon
- ½ cup brown sugar
- 2 tbsp. butter, cold & cut in cubes
- 1 cup powdered sugar

Directions:

1. In a large bowl, add water and sprinkle yeast over top, stir to dissolve.
2. Stir in 1/3 cup milk, egg, and sugar until combined.
3. Add 2 cups flour and stir in until batter gets thick. With a wooden spoon, or mixer with dough hook attached, beat 100 strokes.
4. Fold in oil and salt. Then stir in 1 ¼ cups flour until dough begins to come together.
5. Mix in cinnamon and transfer dough to a lightly floured work surface. Knead for 5 minutes then form into a ball.
6. Use remaining oil to grease a clean bowl and add dough. Cover and let rise 30 minutes.
7. Spray a 9-inch loaf pan with cooking spray.
8. After 30 minutes, punch dough down and divide into 8 equal pieces.
9. Place brown sugar in a shallow bowl and roll dough pieces in it, forming it into balls. Place in prepared pan and sprinkle remaining brown sugar over top.
10. In a small bowl, combine butter and ¼ cup flour until mixture resembles coarse crumbs. Sprinkle over top of bread.
11. Place rack in position 1 of the oven. Set to convection bake on 325°F and set timer for 35 minutes. After 5 minutes, add pan to the rack and bake 30 minutes or until golden brown.
12. Let cool in pan 10 minutes, then invert onto wire rack.
13. In a small bowl, whisk together powdered sugar and milk until smooth. Drizzle over warm bread and serve.
- **Nutrition Info:** Calories 328, Total Fat 6g, Saturated Fat 2g, Total Carbs 60g, Net Carbs 58g, Protein 6g, Sugar 25g, Fiber 2g, Sodium 266mg, Potassium 94mg, Phosphorus 71mg

53. Sweet Potato And Black Bean Burritos

Servings: 6 Burritos
Cooking Time: 30 Minutes
Ingredients:
- 2 sweet potatoes, peeled and cut into a small dice
- 1 tablespoon vegetable oil
- Kosher salt and ground black pepper, to taste
- 6 large flour tortillas
- 1 (16-ounce / 454-g) can refried black beans, divided
- 1½ cups baby spinach, divided
- 6 eggs, scrambled
- ¾ cup grated Cheddar cheese, divided
- ¼ cup salsa
- ¼ cup sour cream
- Cooking spray

Directions:
1. Put the sweet potatoes in a large bowl, then drizzle with vegetable oil and sprinkle with salt and black pepper. Toss to coat well.
2. Place the potatoes in the air fryer basket.
3. Put the air fryer basket on the baking pan and slide into Rack Position 2, select Air Fry, set temperature to 400ºF (205ºC) and set time to 10 minutes.
4. Flip the potatoes halfway through the cooking time.
5. When done, the potatoes should be lightly browned. Remove the potatoes from the oven.
6. Unfold the tortillas on a clean work surface. Divide the black beans, spinach, air fried sweet potatoes, scrambled eggs, and cheese on top of the tortillas.
7. Fold the long side of the tortillas over the filling, then fold in the shorter side to wrap the filling to make the burritos.
8. Wrap the burritos in the aluminum foil and put in the pan.
9. Put the air fryer basket on the baking pan and slide into Rack Position 2, select Air Fry, set temperature to 350ºF (180ºC) and set time to 20 minutes.
10. Flip the burritos halfway through the cooking time.
11. Remove the burritos from the oven and spread with sour cream and salsa. Serve immediately.

54. Fruit Oatmeal With Coconut Flakes

Servings:x
Cooking Time:x
Ingredients:

- 2 cups old fashioned rolled oats
- 1 tsp vanilla extract
- 1 cup blueberries
- 1 cup raspberries
- 1 tsp baking powder
- 2 tsp brown sugar
- ½ tsp cinnamon
- ¼ cup unsweetened coconut flakes
- 2 cups low fat milk
- 2 egg whites

Directions:
1. Preheat oven to 350°F.
2. Combine oats, baking powder, brown sugar, cinnamon and coconut
3. flakes in a greased Breville smart oven.
4. Add milk, egg whites and vanilla and stir well.
5. Add fruits and combine gently so as not to break up fruit.
6. Cook for 30-35 minutes until set and golden brown.

55. Breakfast Oatmeal Cake

Servings: 8
Cooking Time: 25 Minutes
Ingredients:
- 2 eggs
- 1 tbsp coconut oil
- 3 tbsp yogurt
- 1/2 tsp baking powder
- 1 tsp cinnamon
- 1 tsp vanilla
- 3 tbsp honey
- 1/2 tsp baking soda
- 1 apple, peel & chopped
- 1 cup oats

Directions:
1. Fit the Cuisinart oven with the rack in position
2. Line baking dish with parchment paper and set aside.
3. Add 3/4 cup oats and remaining ingredients into the blender and blend until smooth.
4. Add remaining oats and stir well.
5. Pour mixture into the prepared baking dish.
6. Set to bake at 350 F for 30 minutes. After 5 minutes place the baking dish in the preheated oven.

7. Slice and serve.
- **Nutrition Info:** Calories 114 Fat 3.6 g Carbohydrates 18.2 g Sugar 10 g Protein 3.2 g Cholesterol 41 mg

56. Beans And Pork Mix

Servings: 4
Cooking Time: 20 Minutes
Ingredients:
- 1-pound pork stew meat, ground
- 1 red onion, chopped
- 1 tablespoon olive oil
- 1 cup canned kidney beans, drained and rinsed
- 1 teaspoon chili powder
- Salt and black pepper to the taste
- ¼ teaspoon cumin, ground

Directions:
1. Heat up your air fryer at 360 degrees F, add the meat and the onion and cook for 5 minutes.
2. Add the beans and the rest of the ingredients, toss and cook for 15 minutes more.
3. Divide everything into bowls and serve for breakfast.
- **Nutrition Info:** calories 203, fat 4, fiber 6, carbs 12, protein 4

57. Lemon Blueberry Bread

Servings: 12
Cooking Time: 55 Minutes
Ingredients:
- 2 eggs
- 1/4 cup yogurt
- 1/2 cup maple syrup
- 1 tsp baking powder
- 1 3/4 cups all-purpose flour
- 3 tbsp lemon zest, grated
- 3/4 cup blueberries
- 1/4 cup fresh lemon juice
- 1/4 cup coconut oil, melted
- 1/2 tsp salt

Directions:
1. Fit the Cuisinart oven with the rack in position
2. In a bowl, mix all-purpose flour, salt, and baking powder.

3. In a separate bowl, beat eggs with lemon juice, coconut oil, maple syrup, and yogurt.
4. Add flour mixture into the egg mixture and mix until well combined.
5. Add blueberries and lemon zest and stir well.
6. Pour batter into the greased 8*4-inch loaf pan.
7. Set to bake at 350 F for 60 minutes, after 5 minutes, place the loaf pan in the oven.
8. Slice and serve.
- **Nutrition Info:** Calories 162 Fat 5.6 g Carbohydrates 25.1 g Sugar 9.4 g Protein 3.2 g Cholesterol 28 mg

58. Delicious Baked Eggs

Servings: 8
Cooking Time: 45 Minutes
Ingredients:
- 12 eggs
- 1/2 cup all-purpose flour
- 16 oz cottage cheese
- 16 oz cheddar cheese, shredded
- 1 tsp salt

Directions:
1. Fit the Cuisinart oven with the rack in position
2. Grease 9*13-inch baking pan with butter and set aside.
3. In a large bowl, whisk eggs with flour, cottage cheese, cheddar cheese, and salt.
4. Pour egg mixture into the prepared baking pan.
5. Set to bake at 350 F for 50 minutes. After 5 minutes place the baking pan in the preheated oven.
6. Serve and enjoy.
- **Nutrition Info:** Calories 402 Fat 26.5 g Carbohydrates 9.3 g Sugar 1 g Protein 31 g Cholesterol 310 mg

59. Spinach Egg Breakfast

Servings: 4
Cooking Time: 20 Minutes
Ingredients:
- 3 eggs
- 1/4 cup coconut milk

- 1/4 cup parmesan cheese, grated 4 oz spinach, chopped
- 3 oz cottage cheese

Directions:
1. Preheat the air fryer to 350 F.
2. Add eggs, milk, half parmesan cheese, and cottage cheese in a bowl and whisk well. Add spinach and stir well.
3. Pour mixture into the air fryer baking dish.
4. Sprinkle remaining half parmesan cheese on top.
5. Place dish in the air fryer and cook for 20 minutes.
6. Serve and enjoy.
- **Nutrition Info:** Calories 144 Fat 8.5 g Carbohydrates 2.5 g Sugar 1.1 g Protein 14 g Cholesterol 135 mg

60. Crustless Broccoli Quiche

Servings:4
Cooking Time: 10 Minutes
Ingredients:
- 1 cup broccoli florets
- ¾ cup chopped roasted red peppers
- 1¼ cups grated Fontina cheese
- 6 eggs
- ¾ cup heavy cream
- ½ teaspoon salt
- Freshly ground black pepper, to taste
- Cooking spray

Directions:
1. Spritz the baking pan with cooking spray
2. Add the broccoli florets and roasted red peppers to the pan and scatter the grated Fontina cheese on top.
3. In a bowl, beat together the eggs and heavy cream. Sprinkle with salt and pepper. Pour the egg mixture over the top of the cheese. Wrap the pan in foil.
4. Put the air fryer basket on the baking pan and slide into Rack Position 2, select Air Fry, set temperature to 325ºF (163ºC) and set time to 10 minutes.
5. After 8 minutes, remove the pan from the oven. Remove the foil. Return to the oven and continue to cook for another 2 minutes.
6. When cooked, the quiche should be golden brown.

7. Rest for 5 minutes before cutting into wedges and serve warm.

61. Creamy Mushroom And Spinach Omelet

Servings: 2
Cooking Time: 10 Minutes
Ingredients:
- 4 eggs, lightly beaten
- 2 tbsp heavy cream
- 2 cups spinach, chopped
- 1 cup mushrooms, chopped
- 3 oz feta cheese, crumbled
- 1 tbsp fresh parsley, chopped
- Salt and black pepper to taste

Directions:
1. Spray a baking pan with cooking spray. In a bowl, whisk eggs and heavy cream until combined. Stir in spinach, mushrooms, feta, salt, and pepper.
2. Pour into the basket tray and cook in your Cuisinart for 6-10 minutes at 350 F on Bake function until golden and set. Sprinkle with parsley, cut into wedges, and serve.

62. Cinnamon Mango Bread

Servings: 4
Cooking Time: 60 Minutes
Ingredients:
- ½ cup melted butter
- 1 egg, lightly beaten
- ½ cup brown sugar
- 1 tsp vanilla extract
- 3 ripe mango, mashed
- 1 ½ cups plain flour
- 1 tsp baking powder
- ½ tsp grated nutmeg
- ½ tsp ground cinnamon

Directions:
1. Spray the Cuisinart baking pan with cooking spray and line with parchment paper. In a bowl, whisk butter, egg, sugar, vanilla, and mango. Sift in flour, baking powder, nutmeg, and cinnamon and stir without overmixing. Pour the batter into the pan and place in the toaster oven.
2. Cook for 25-30 minutes at 360 F on Bake function until a toothpick inserted in the

middle comes out clean. Let cool on a wire rack before slicing. Serve.

63. Buttered Apple & Brie Cheese Sandwich

Servings: 1
Cooking Time: 10 Minutes
Ingredients:
- 2 bread slices
- ½ apple, thinly sliced
- 2 tsp butter
- 2 oz brie cheese, thinly sliced

Directions:
1. Spread butter on the bread slices. Top with apple slices. Place brie slices on top of the apples. Finish with the other slice of bread. Cook in Cuisinart for 5 minutes at 350 F on Bake function.

64. Air Fried Cream Cheese Wontons

Servings:4
Cooking Time: 6 Minutes
Ingredients:
- 2 ounces (57 g) cream cheese, softened
- 1 tablespoon sugar
- 16 square wonton wrappers
- Cooking spray

Directions:
1. Spritz the air fryer basket with cooking spray.
2. In a mixing bowl, stir together the cream cheese and sugar until well mixed. Prepare a small bowl of water alongside.
3. On a clean work surface, lay the wonton wrappers. Scoop ¼ teaspoon of cream cheese in the center of each wonton wrapper. Dab the water over the wrapper edges. Fold each wonton wrapper diagonally in half over the filling to form a triangle.
4. Arrange the wontons in the pan. Spritz the wontons with cooking spray.
5. Put the air fryer basket on the baking pan and slide into Rack Position 2, select Air Fry, set temperature to 350ºF (180ºC) and set time to 6 minutes.
6. Flip the wontons halfway through the cooking time.

7. When cooking is complete, the wontons will be golden brown and crispy.
8. Divide the wontons among four plates. Let rest for 5 minutes before serving.

65. Cheddar Eggs With Potatoes

Servings:3
Cooking Time: 24 Minutes
Ingredients:

- 3 potatoes, thinly sliced
- 2 eggs, beaten
- 2 oz cheddar cheese, shredded
- 1 tbsp all-purpose flour
- ½ cup coconut cream

Directions:

1. Preheat Breville on AirFry function to 390 F. Place the potatoes the basket and press Start. Cook for 12 minutes. Mix the eggs, coconut cream, and flour until the cream mixture thickens.
2. Remove the potatoes from the oven, line them in the ramekin and top with the cream mixture. Top with the cheddar cheese. Cook for 12 more minutes.

66. Breakfast Egg Tomato

Servings: 2
Cooking Time: 24 Minutes
Ingredients:

- 2 eggs
- 2 large fresh tomatoes 1 tsp fresh parsley Pepper
- Salt

Directions:

1. Preheat the air fryer to 325 F.
2. Cut off the top of a tomato and spoon out the tomato innards.
3. Break the egg in each tomato and place in air fryer basket and cook for 24 minutes.
4. Season with parsley, pepper, and salt.
5. Serve and enjoy.
- **Nutrition Info:** Calories 95 Fat 5 g Carbohydrates 7.5 g Sugar 5.1 g Protein 7 g Cholesterol 164 mg

67. Mini Cinnamon Rolls

Servings: 18 Rolls
Cooking Time: 25 Minutes

Ingredients:

- $^1/_3$ cup light brown sugar
- 2 teaspoons cinnamon
- 1 (9-by-9-inch) frozen puff pastry sheet, thawed
- All-purpose flour, for dusting
- 6 teaspoons unsalted butter, melted, divided

Directions:

1. In a small bowl, stir together the brown sugar and cinnamon.
2. On a clean work surface, lightly dust with the flour and lay the puff pastry sheet. Using a rolling pin, press the folds together and roll the dough out in one direction so that it measures about 9 by 11 inches. Cut it in half to form two squat rectangles of about 5½ by 9 inches.
3. Brush 2 teaspoons of the butter over each pastry half. Sprinkle with 2 tablespoons of the cinnamon sugar. Pat it down lightly with the palm of your hand to help it adhere to the butter.
4. Starting with the 9-inch side of one rectangle. Using your hands, carefully roll the dough into a cylinder. Repeat with the other rectangle. To make slicing easier, refrigerate the rolls for 10 to 20 minutes.
5. Using a sharp knife, slice each roll into nine 1-inch pieces. Transfer the rolls to the center of the baking pan. They should be very close to each other, but not quite touching. Drizzle the remaining 2 teaspoons of the butter over the rolls and sprinkle with the remaining cinnamon sugar.
6. Slide the baking pan into Rack Position 1, select Convection Bake, set temperature to 350ºF (180ºC) and set time to 25 minutes.
7. When cooking is complete, remove the pan and check the rolls. They should be puffed up and golden brown.
8. Let the rolls rest for 5 minutes and transfer them to a wire rack to cool completely. Serve.

68. Tator Tots Casserole

Servings: 8
Cooking Time: 30 Minutes

Ingredients:

- 8 eggs
- 28 oz tator tots
- 8 oz pepper jack cheese, shredded
- 2 green onions, sliced
- 1/4 cup milk
- 1 lb breakfast sausage, cooked
- Pepper
- Salt

Directions:

1. Fit the Cuisinart oven with the rack in position
2. Spray 13*9-inch baking pan with cooking spray and set aside.
3. In a bowl, whisk eggs with milk, pepper, and salt.
4. Layer sausage in a prepared baking pan then pour the egg mixture and sprinkle with half shredded cheese and green onions.
5. Add tator tots on top.
6. Set to bake at 400 F for 35 minutes. After 5 minutes place the baking pan in the preheated oven.
7. Top with remaining cheese and serve.
- **Nutrition Info:** Calories 398 Fat 31.5 g Carbohydrates 2 g Sugar 0.8 g Protein 22.1 g Cholesterol 251 mg

69. Veggie Frittata

Servings:4
Cooking Time: 12 Minutes
Ingredients:

- ½ cup chopped red bell pepper
- $^1/_3$ cup grated carrot
- $^1/_3$ cup minced onion
- 1 teaspoon olive oil
- 1 egg
- 6 egg whites
- $^1/_3$ cup 2% milk
- 1 tablespoon shredded Parmesan cheese

Directions:

1. Mix together the red bell pepper, carrot, onion, and olive oil in the baking pan and stir to combine.
2. Slide the baking pan into Rack Position 1, select Convection Bake, set temperature to 350ºF (180ºC) and set time to 12 minutes.

3. After 3 minutes, remove the pan from the oven. Stir the vegetables. Return the pan to the oven and continue cooking.
4. Meantime, whisk together the egg, egg whites, and milk in a medium bowl until creamy.
5. After 3 minutes, remove the pan from the oven. Pour the egg mixture over the top and scatter with the Parmesan cheese. Return the pan to the oven and continue cooking for additional 6 minutes.
6. When cooking is complete, the eggs will be set and the top will be golden around the edges.
7. Allow the frittata to cool for 5 minutes before slicing and serving.

70. Easy Buttermilk Biscuits

Servings: 16 Biscuits
Cooking Time: 18 Minutes
Ingredients:

- 2½ cups all-purpose flour
- 1 tablespoon baking powder
- 1 teaspoon kosher salt
- 1 teaspoon sugar
- ½ teaspoon baking soda
- 8 tablespoons (1 stick) unsalted butter, at room temperature
- 1 cup buttermilk, chilled

Directions:

1. Stir together the flour, baking powder, salt, sugar, and baking powder in a large bowl.
2. Add the butter and stir to mix well. Pour in the buttermilk and stir with a rubber spatula just until incorporated.
3. Place the dough onto a lightly floured surface and roll the dough out to a disk, ½ inch thick. Cut out the biscuits with a 2-inch round cutter and re-roll any scraps until you have 16 biscuits. Arrange the biscuits in the baking pan.
4. Slide the baking pan into Rack Position 1, select Convection Bake, set temperature to 325ºF (163ºC) and set time to 18 minutes.
5. When cooked, the biscuits will be golden brown.
6. Remove from the oven to a plate and serve hot.

71. Maple Walnut Pancake

Servings:4
Cooking Time: 20 Minutes
Ingredients:

- 3 tablespoons melted butter, divided
- 1 cup flour
- 2 tablespoons sugar
- 1½ teaspoons baking powder
- ¼ teaspoon salt
- 1 egg, beaten
- ¾ cup milk
- 1 teaspoon pure vanilla extract
- ½ cup roughly chopped walnuts
- Maple syrup or fresh sliced fruit, for serving

Directions:

1. Grease the baking pan with 1 tablespoon of melted butter.
2. Mix together the flour, sugar, baking powder, and salt in a medium bowl. Add the beaten egg, milk, the remaining 2 tablespoons of melted butter, and vanilla and stir until the batter is sticky but slightly lumpy.
3. Slowly pour the batter into the greased baking pan and scatter with the walnuts.
4. Slide the baking pan into Rack Position 1, select Convection Bake, set temperature to 330ºF (166ºC) and set time to 20 minutes.
5. When cooked, the pancake should be golden brown and cooked through.
6. Let the pancake rest for 5 minutes and serve topped with the maple syrup or fresh fruit, if desired.

72. Parsley Sausage Patties

Servings:4
Cooking Time: 20 Minutes
Ingredients:

- 1 lb ground Italian sausage
- ¼ cup breadcrumbs
- 1 tsp dried parsley
- 1 tsp red pepper flakes
- Salt and black pepper to taste
- ¼ tsp garlic powder
- 1 egg, beaten

Directions:

1. Preheat Breville on Bake function to 350 F. Line a baking sheet with parchment paper. Combine all the ingredients in a large bowl.
2. Make patties out of the sausage mixture and arrange them on the baking sheet. Press Start. Cook for 15 minutes until golden.

73. Lemon Vanilla Cupcakes With Yogurt Frost

Servings: 4
Cooking Time: 25 Minutes
Ingredients:

- Lemon Frosting:
- 1 cup natural yogurt
- 2 tbsp sugar
- 1 orange, juiced
- 1 tbsp orange zest
- 7 oz cream cheese, softened
- Cupcake:
- 2 lemons, seeded and quartered
- ½ cup flour + extra for basing
- ¼ tsp salt
- 2 tbsp sugar
- 1 tsp baking powder
- 1 tsp vanilla extract
- 2 eggs
- ½ cup butter, softened
- 2 tbsp milk

Directions:

1. In a bowl, add the yogurt and cream cheese. Mix until smooth. Add in the orange juice and zest; mix well. Gradually add the sugar while stirring until smooth. Make sure the frost is not runny. Set aside.
2. Place the lemon quarters in a food processor and process it until pureed. Add the flour, baking powder, butter, milk, eggs, vanilla extract, sugar, and salt. Process again until smooth.
3. Preheat Cuisinart on Bake function to 360 F. Flour the bottom of 8 cupcake cases and spoon the batter into the cases ¾ way up. Place them in the Air Fryer tray and bake for 8-12 minutes. Once ready, remove and let cool. Design the cupcakes with the frosting and serve.

74. Flavorful Zucchini Frittata

Servings: 4
Cooking Time: 25 Minutes
Ingredients:

- 6 eggs
- 2 cups zucchini, grated & squeeze out excess liquid
- 1 cup cheddar cheese, shredded
- 1 cup ham, chopped
- 1/4 cup heavy cream
- 2 tbsp butter
- 1/4 tsp pepper
- 1 tsp salt

Directions:

1. Fit the Cuisinart oven with the rack in position
2. Melt butter in a pan over medium heat.
3. Add zucchini in the pan and sauté until tender. Remove pan from heat.
4. In a bowl, whisk eggs and cream. Stir in zucchini, cheese, ham, pepper, and salt.
5. Pour mixture into the greased baking dish.
6. Set to bake at 325 F for 30 minutes. After 5 minutes place the baking dish in the preheated oven.
7. Serve and enjoy.
- **Nutrition Info:** Calories 349 Fat 27.5 g Carbohydrates 4.3 g Sugar 1.7 g Protein 21.8 gCholesterol 320 mg

75. Breakfast Oatmeal With Blueberries

Servings:x
Cooking Time:x
Ingredients:

- 1-2 Tbsp butter
- ½ Gala apple, peeled, cored and cut into ½-inch pieces
- Pinch kosher salt
- ⅔ cup whole milk
- 1 egg yolk
- ½ cup fresh blueberries
- 1 Tbsp maple syrup
- ⅔ cup uncooked rolled oats
- ¼ cup blanched slivered almonds
- ¼ tsp baking powder
- ¼ tsp cinnamon
- 2 tsp brown sugar

- ¼ tsp vanilla extract

Directions:

1. Preheat the oven to 375°F.
2. Butter the bottom of Breville smart oven and about 1 inch up the sides.
3. Add the apple and blueberries in a thin layer. Drizzle with the maple syrup.
4. In a medium bowl, mix together the oats, almonds, baking powder, cinnamon, and salt.
5. In a small bowl, whisk together the milk, egg yolk, sugar, and vanilla and pour over the oat mixture. Stir just until combined and spoon over the fruit.
6. Bake, uncovered, for 30 to 35 minutes, or until the top is golden brown and the fruit is bubbling. Let cool for 10 to 15 minutes before serving.

76. Feta & Spinach Omelet With Mushrooms

Servings:2
Cooking Time: 10 Minutes
Ingredients:

- 4 eggs, lightly beaten
- 2 tbsp heavy cream
- 2 cups spinach, chopped
- 1 cup mushrooms, chopped
- 3 oz feta cheese, crumbled
- A handful of fresh parsley, chopped
- Salt and black pepper to taste

Directions:

1. In a bowl, whisk eggs and stir in spinach, mushrooms, feta, parsley, salt, and pepper. Pour into a greased baking pan and cook in the Breville oven for 12-14 minutes at 350 F on Bake function..

77. Strawberries And Quinoa Salad

Servings: 4
Cooking Time: 15 Minutes
Ingredients:

- 1 cup strawberries
- 1 cup quinoa, cooked
- 1 cup coconut milk
- ½ cup heavy cream
- 2 tablespoons sugar
- Cooking spray

Directions:

1. Grease your air fryer with cooking spray, and combine the berries with the milk, quinoa, cream and sugar inside.
2. Toss, cook at 365 degrees F for 15 minutes, divide into bowls and serve for breakfast.
- **Nutrition Info:** calories 172, fat 6, fiber 8, carbs 11, protein 5

78. Air Fried Philly Cheesesteaks

Servings:2
Cooking Time: 20 Minutes
Ingredients:

- 12 ounces (340 g) boneless rib-eye steak, sliced thinly
- ½ teaspoon Worcestershire sauce
- ½ teaspoon soy sauce
- Kosher salt and ground black pepper, to taste
- ½ green bell pepper, stemmed, deseeded, and thinly sliced
- ½ small onion, halved and thinly sliced
- 1 tablespoon vegetable oil
- 2 soft hoagie rolls, split three-fourths of the way through
- 1 tablespoon butter, softened
- 2 slices provolone cheese, halved

Directions:

1. Combine the steak, Worcestershire sauce, soy sauce, salt, and ground black pepper in a large bowl. Toss to coat well. Set aside.
2. Combine the bell pepper, onion, salt, ground black pepper, and vegetable oil in a separate bowl. Toss to coat the vegetables well.
3. Place the steak and vegetables in the air fryer basket.
4. Put the air fryer basket on the baking pan and slide into Rack Position 2, select Air Fry, set temperature to 400ºF (205ºC) and set time to 15 minutes.
5. When cooked, the steak will be browned and vegetables will be tender. Transfer them onto a plate. Set aside.
6. Brush the hoagie rolls with butter and place in the basket.
7. Select Toast and set time to 3 minutes. Return to the oven. When done, the rolls should be lightly browned.
8. Transfer the rolls to a clean work surface and divide the steak and vegetable mix between the rolls. Spread with cheese. Transfer the stuffed rolls to the basket.
9. Select Air Fry and set time to 2 minutes. Return to the oven. When done, the cheese should be melted.
10. Serve immediately.

LUNCH RECIPES

79. Turkey Meatballs With Manchego Cheese

Servings: 4
Cooking Time: 10 Minutes
Ingredients:

- 1 pound ground turkey
- 1/2 pound ground pork
- 1 egg, well beaten
- 1 teaspoon dried basil
- 1 teaspoon dried rosemary
- 1/4 cup Manchego cheese, grated
- 2 tablespoons yellow onions, finely chopped
- 1 teaspoon fresh garlic, finely chopped
- Sea salt and ground black pepper, to taste

Directions:

1. In a mixing bowl, combine all the ingredients until everything is well incorporated.
2. Shape the mixture into 1-inch balls.
3. Cook the meatballs in the preheated Air Fryer at 380 degrees for 7 minutes. Shake halfway through the cooking time. Work in batches.
4. Serve with your favorite pasta.
- **Nutrition Info:** 386 Calories; 24g Fat; 9g Carbs; 41g Protein; 3g Sugars; 2g Fiber

80. Beef Steaks With Beans

Servings: 4
Cooking Time: 10 Minutes
Ingredients:

- 4 beef steaks, trim the fat and cut into strips
- 1 cup green onions, chopped
- 2 cloves garlic, minced
- 1 red bell pepper, seeded and thinly sliced
- 1 can tomatoes, crushed
- 1 can cannellini beans
- 3/4 cup beef broth
- 1/4 teaspoon dried basil
- 1/2 teaspoon cayenne pepper
- 1/2 teaspoon sea salt
- 1/4 teaspoon ground black pepper, or to taste

Directions:

1. Preparing the ingredients. Add the steaks, green onions and garlic to the instant crisp air fryer basket.
2. Air frying. Close air fryer lid. Cook at 390 degrees f for 10 minutes, working in batches.
3. Stir in the remaining ingredients and cook for an additional 5 minutes.
- **Nutrition Info:** Calories 284 Total fat 7.9 g Saturated fat 1.4 g Cholesterol 36 mg Sodium 704 mg Total carbs 46 g Fiber 3.6 g Sugar 5.5 g Protein 17.9 g

81. Barbecue Air Fried Chicken

Servings: 10
Cooking Time: 26 Minutes
Ingredients:

- 1 teaspoon Liquid Smoke
- 2 cloves Fresh Garlic smashed
- 1/2 cup Apple Cider Vinegar
- 3 pounds Chuck Roast well-marbled with intramuscular fat
- 1 Tablespoon Kosher Salt
- 1 Tablespoon Freshly Ground Black Pepper
- 2 teaspoons Garlic Powder
- 1.5 cups Barbecue Sauce
- 1/4 cup Light Brown Sugar + more for sprinkling
- 2 Tablespoons Honey optional and in place of 2 TBL sugar

Directions:

1. Add meat to the Instant Pot Duo Crisp Air Fryer Basket, spreading out the meat.
2. Select the option Air Fry.
3. Close the Air Fryer lid and cook at 300 degrees F for 8 minutes. Pause the Air Fryer and flip meat over after 4 minutes.
4. Remove the lid and baste with more barbecue sauce and sprinkle with a little brown sugar.
5. Again Close the Air Fryer lid and set the temperature at 400°F for 9 minutes. Watch meat though the lid and flip it over after 5 minutes.
- **Nutrition Info:** Calories 360, Total Fat 16g, Total Carbs 27g, Protein 27g

82. Spanish Chicken Bake

Servings: 4
Cooking Time: 25 Minutes
Ingredients:

- ½ onion, quartered
- ½ red onion, quartered
- ½ lb. potatoes, quartered
- 4 garlic cloves
- 4 tomatoes, quartered
- 1/8 cup chorizo
- ¼ teaspoon paprika powder
- 4 chicken thighs, boneless
- ¼ teaspoon dried oregano
- ½ green bell pepper, julienned
- Salt
- Black pepper

Directions:

1. Toss chicken, veggies, and all the Ingredients: in a baking tray.
2. Press "Power Button" of Air Fry Oven and turn the dial to select the "Bake" mode.
3. Press the Time button and again turn the dial to set the cooking time to 25 minutes.
4. Now push the Temp button and rotate the dial to set the temperature at 425 degrees F.
5. Once preheated, place the baking pan inside and close its lid.
6. Serve warm.
- **Nutrition Info:** Calories 301 Total Fat 8.9 g Saturated Fat 4.5 g Cholesterol 57 mg Sodium 340 mg Total Carbs 24.7 g Fiber 1.2 g Sugar 1.3 g Protein 15.3 g

83. Fried Chicken Tacos

Servings: 4
Cooking Time: 10 Minutes
Ingredients:

- Chicken
- 1 lb. chicken tenders or breast chopped into 2-inch pieces
- 1 tsp garlic powder
- ½ tsp onion powder
- 1 large egg
- 1 ½ tsp salt
- 1 tsp paprika
- 3 Tbsp buttermilk
- ¾ cup All-purpose flour
- 3 Tbsp corn starch
- ½ tsp black pepper
- ½ tsp cayenne pepper
- oil for spraying
- Coleslaw
- ¼ tsp red pepper flakes
- 2 cups coleslaw mix
- 1 Tbsp brown sugar
- ½ tsp salt
- 2 Tbsp apple cider vinegar
- 1 Tbsp water
- Spicy Mayo
- ½ tsp salt
- ¼ cup mayonnaise
- 1 tsp garlic powder
- 2 Tbsp hot sauce
- 1 Tbsp buttermilk
- Tortilla wrappers

Directions:

1. Take a large bowl and mix together coleslaw mix, water, brown sugar, salt, apple cider vinegar, and red pepper flakes. Set aside.
2. Take another small bowl and combine mayonnaise, hot sauce, buttermilk, garlic powder, and salt. Set this mixture aside.
3. Select the Instant Pot Duo Crisp Air Fryer option, adjust the temperature to 360°F and push start. Preheating will start.
4. Create a clear station by placing two large flat pans side by side. Whisk together egg and buttermilk with salt and pepper in one of them. In the second, whisk flour, corn starch, black pepper, garlic powder, onion powder, salt, paprika, and cayenne pepper.
5. Cut the chicken tenders into 1-inch pieces. Season all pieces with a little salt and pepper.
6. Once the Instant Pot Duo Crisp Air Fryer is preheated, remove the tray and lightly spray it with oil. Coat your chicken with egg mixture while shaking off any excess egg, followed by the flour mixture, and place it on the tray and tray in the basket, making sure your chicken pieces don't overlap.
7. Close the Air Fryer lid, and cook on 360°F for 10 minutes

8. while flipping and spraying halfway through cooking.
9. Once the chicken is done, remove and place chicken into warmed tortilla shells. Top with coleslaw and spicy mayonnaise.
- **Nutrition Info:** Calories 375, Total Fat 15g, Total Carbs 31g, Protein 29g

84. Chicken Potato Bake

Servings: 4
Cooking Time: 25 Minutes
Ingredients:
- 4 potatoes, diced
- 1 tablespoon garlic, minced
- 1.5 tablespoons olive oil
- 1/8 teaspoon salt
- 1/8 teaspoon pepper
- 1.5 lbs. boneless skinless chicken
- 3/4 cup mozzarella cheese, shredded
- parsley chopped

Directions:
1. Toss chicken and potatoes with all the spices and oil in a baking pan.
2. Drizzle the cheese on top of the chicken and potato.
3. Press "Power Button" of Air Fry Oven and turn the dial to select the "Bake" mode.
4. Press the Time button and again turn the dial to set the cooking time to 25 minutes.
5. Now push the Temp button and rotate the dial to set the temperature at 375 degrees F.
6. Once preheated, place the baking pan inside and close its lid.
7. Serve warm.
- **Nutrition Info:** Calories 695 Total Fat 17.5 g Saturated Fat 4.8 g Cholesterol 283 mg Sodium 355 mg Total Carbs 26.4 g Fiber 1.8 g Sugar 0.8 g Protein 117.4 g

85. Crispy Breaded Pork Chop

Servings: 6
Cooking Time: 12 Minutes
Ingredients:
- olive oil spray
- 6 3/4-inch thick center-cut boneless pork chops, fat trimmed (5 oz each)
- kosher salt
- 1 large egg, beaten

- 1/2 cup panko crumbs, check labels for GF
- 1/3 cup crushed cornflakes crumbs
- 2 tbsp grated parmesan cheese
- 1 1/4 tsp sweet paprika
- 1/2 tsp garlic powder
- 1/2 tsp onion powder
- 1/4 tsp chili powder
- 1/8 tsp black pepper

Directions:
1. Preheat the Instant Pot Duo Crisp Air Fryer for 12 minutes at 400°F.
2. On both sides, season pork chops with half teaspoon kosher salt.
3. Then combine cornflake crumbs, panko, parmesan cheese, 3/4 tsp kosher salt, garlic powder, paprika, onion powder, chili powder, and black pepper in a large bowl.
4. Place the egg beat in another bowl. Dip the pork in the egg & then crumb mixture.
5. When the air fryer is ready, place 3 of the chops into the Instant Pot Duo Crisp Air Fryer Basket and spritz the top with oil.
6. Close the Air Fryer lid and cook for 12 minutes turning halfway, spritzing both sides with oil.
7. Set aside and repeat with the remaining.
- **Nutrition Info:** Calories 281, Total Fat 13g, Total Carbs 8g, Protein 33g

86. Orange Chicken Rice

Servings: 4
Cooking Time: 55 Minutes
Ingredients:
- 3 tablespoons olive oil
- 1 medium onion, chopped
- 1 3/4 cups chicken broth
- 1 cup brown basmati rice
- Zest and juice of 2 oranges
- Salt to taste
- 4 (6-oz.) boneless, skinless chicken thighs
- Black pepper, to taste
- 2 tablespoons fresh mint, chopped
- 2 tablespoons pine nuts, toasted

Directions:
1. Spread the rice in a casserole dish and place the chicken on top.
2. Toss the rest of the Ingredients: in a bowl and liberally pour over the chicken.

3. Press "Power Button" of Air Fry Oven and turn the dial to select the "Bake" mode.
4. Press the Time button and again turn the dial to set the cooking time to 55 minutes.
5. Now push the Temp button and rotate the dial to set the temperature at 350 degrees F.
6. Once preheated, place the casserole dish inside and close its lid.
7. Serve warm.
- **Nutrition Info:** Calories 231 Total Fat 20.1 g Saturated Fat 2.4 g Cholesterol 110 mg Sodium 941 mg Total Carbs 30.1 g Fiber 0.9 g Sugar 1.4 g Protein 14.6 g

87. Roasted Stuffed Peppers

Servings: 4
Cooking Time: 20 Minutes
Ingredients:
- 4 ounces shredded cheddar cheese
- ½ tsp. Pepper
- ½ tsp. Salt
- 1 tsp. Worcestershire sauce
- ½ c. Tomato sauce
- 8 ounces lean ground beef
- 1 tsp. Olive oil
- 1 minced garlic clove
- ½ chopped onion
- 2 green peppers

Directions:
1. Preparing the ingredients. Ensure your instant crisp air fryer is preheated to 390 degrees. Spray with olive oil.
2. Cut stems off bell peppers and remove seeds. Cook in boiling salted water for 3 minutes.
3. Sauté garlic and onion together in a skillet until golden in color.
4. Take skillet off the heat. Mix pepper, salt, Worcestershire sauce, ¼ cup of tomato sauce, half of cheese and beef together.
5. Divide meat mixture into pepper halves. Top filled peppers with remaining cheese and tomato sauce.
6. Place filled peppers in the instant crisp air fryer.
7. Air frying. Close air fryer lid. Set temperature to 390°f, and set time to 20 minutes, bake 15-20 minutes.

- **Nutrition Info:** Calories: 295; Fat: 8g; Protein:23g; Sugar:2g

88. Okra Casserole

Servings: 4
Cooking Time: 12 Minutes
Ingredients:
- 2 red bell peppers; cubed
- 2 tomatoes; chopped.
- 3 garlic cloves; minced
- 3 cups okra
- ½ cup cheddar; shredded
- ¼ cup tomato puree
- 1 tbsp. cilantro; chopped.
- 1 tsp. olive oil
- 2 tsp. coriander, ground
- Salt and black pepper to taste.

Directions:
1. Grease a heat proof dish that fits your air fryer with the oil, add all the ingredients except the cilantro and the cheese and toss them really gently
2. Sprinkle the cheese and the cilantro on top, introduce the dish in the fryer and cook at 390°F for 20 minutes.
3. Divide between plates and serve for lunch.
- **Nutrition Info:** Calories: 221; Fat: 7g; Fiber: 2g; Carbs: 4g; Protein: 9g

89. Fried Paprika Tofu

Servings:
Cooking Time: 12 Minutes
Ingredients:
- 1 block extra firm tofu; pressed to remove excess water and cut into cubes
- 1/4 cup cornstarch
- 1 tablespoon smoked paprika
- salt and pepper to taste

Directions:
1. Line the Air Fryer basket with aluminum foil and brush with oil. Preheat the Air Fryer to 370 - degrees Fahrenheit.
2. Mix all ingredients in a bowl. Toss to combine. Place in the Air Fryer basket and cook for 12 minutes.

90. Sweet Potato And Parsnip Spiralized Latkes

Servings: 12
Cooking Time: 20 Minutes
Ingredients:

- 1 medium sweet potato
- 1 large parsnip
- 4 cups water
- 1 egg + 1 egg white
- 2 scallions
- 1/2 teaspoon garlic powder
- 1/2 teaspoon sea salt
- 1/2 teaspoon ground pepper

Directions:

1. Start by spiralizing the sweet potato and parsnip and chopping the scallions, reserving only the green parts.
2. Preheat toaster oven to 425°F.
3. Bring 4 cups of water to a boil. Place all of your noodles in a colander and pour the boiling water over the top, draining well.
4. Let the noodles cool, then grab handfuls and place them in a paper towel; squeeze to remove as much liquid as possible.
5. In a large bowl, beat egg and egg white together. Add noodles, scallions, garlic powder, salt, and pepper, mix well.
6. Prepare a baking sheet; scoop out 1/4 cup of mixture at a time and place on sheet.
7. Slightly press down each scoop with your hands, then bake for 20 minutes, flipping halfway through.
- **Nutrition Info:** Calories: 24, Sodium: 91 mg, Dietary Fiber: 1.0 g, Total Fat: 0.4 g, Total Carbs: 4.3 g, Protein: 0.9 g.

91. Chicken With Veggies And Rice

Servings: 3
Cooking Time: 20 Minutes
Ingredients:

- 3 cups cold boiled white rice
- 1 cup cooked chicken, diced
- ½ cup frozen carrots
- ½ cup frozen peas
- ½ cup onion, chopped
- 6 tablespoons soy sauce
- 1 tablespoon vegetable oil

Directions:

1. Preheat the Air fryer to 360 degree F and grease a 7" nonstick pan.
2. Mix the rice, soy sauce, and vegetable oil in a bowl.
3. Stir in the remaining ingredients and mix until well combined.
4. Transfer the rice mixture into the pan and place in the Air fryer.
5. Cook for about 20 minutes and dish out to serve immediately.
- **Nutrition Info:** Calories: 405, Fat: 6.4g, Carbohydrates: 63g, Sugar: 3.5g, Protein: 21.7g, Sodium: 1500mg

92. Glazed Lamb Chops

Servings: 4
Cooking Time: 15 Minutes
Ingredients:

- 1 tablespoon Dijon mustard
- ½ tablespoon fresh lime juice
- 1 teaspoon honey
- ½ teaspoon olive oil
- Salt and ground black pepper, as required
- 4 (4-ounce) lamb loin chops

Directions:

1. In a black pepper large bowl, mix together the mustard, lemon juice, oil, honey, salt, and black pepper.
2. Add the chops and coat with the mixture generously.
3. Place the chops onto the greased "Sheet Pan".
4. Press "Power Button" of Ninja Foodi Digital Air Fry Oven and turn the dial to select the "Air Bake" mode.
5. Press the Time button and again turn the dial to set the cooking time to 15 minutes.
6. Now push the Temp button and rotate the dial to set the temperature at 390 degrees F.
7. Press "Start/Pause" button to start.
8. When the unit beeps to show that it is preheated, open the lid.
9. Insert the "Sheet Pan" in oven.
10. Flip the chops once halfway through.
11. Serve hot.
- **Nutrition Info:** Calories: 224 kcal Total Fat: 9.1 g Saturated Fat: 3.1 g Cholesterol: 102

mg Sodium: 169 mg Total Carbs: 1.7 g Fiber: 0.1 g Sugar: 1.5 g Protein: 32 g

93. Sweet & Sour Pork

Servings: 4
Cooking Time: 27 Minutes
Ingredients:
- 2 pounds Pork cut into chunks
- 2 large Eggs
- 1 teaspoon Pure Sesame Oil (optional)
- 1 cup Potato Starch (or cornstarch)
- 1/2 teaspoon Sea Salt
- 1/4 teaspoon Freshly Ground Black Pepper
- 1/16 teaspoon Chinese Five Spice
- 3 Tablespoons Canola Oil
- Oil Mister

Directions:
1. In a mixing bowl, combine salt, potato starch, Chinese Five Spice, and peppers.
2. In another bowl, beat the eggs & add sesame oil.
3. Then dredge the pieces of Pork into the Potato Starch and remove the excess. Then dip each piece into the egg mixture, shake off excess, and then back into the Potato Starch mixture.
4. Place pork pieces into the Instant Pot Duo Crisp Air Fryer Basket after spray the pork with oil.
5. Close the Air Fryer lid and cook at 340°F for approximately 8 to12 minutes (or until pork is cooked), shaking the basket a couple of times for evenly distribution.
- **Nutrition Info:** Calories 521, Total Fat 21g, Total Carbs 23g, Protein 60g

94. Duck Rolls

Servings: 3
Cooking Time: 40 Minutes
Ingredients:
- 1 pound duck breast fillet, each cut into 2 pieces
- 3 tablespoons fresh parsley, finely chopped
- 1 small red onion, finely chopped
- 1 garlic clove, crushed
- 1½ teaspoons ground cumin
- 1 teaspoon ground cinnamon
- ½ teaspoon red chili powder
- Salt, to taste
- 2 tablespoons olive oil

Directions:
1. Preheat the Air fryer to 355 degree F and grease an Air fryer basket.
2. Mix the garlic, parsley, onion, spices, and 1 tablespoon of olive oil in a bowl.
3. Make a slit in each duck piece horizontally and coat with onion mixture.
4. Roll each duck piece tightly and transfer into the Air fryer basket.
5. Cook for about 40 minutes and cut into desired size slices to serve.
- **Nutrition Info:** Calories: 239, Fats: 8.2g, Carbohydrates: 3.2g, Sugar: 0.9g, Proteins: 37.5g, Sodium: 46mg

95. Greek Lamb Meatballs

Servings: 12
Cooking Time: 12 Minutes
Ingredients:
- 1 pound ground lamb
- ½ cup breadcrumbs
- ¼ cup milk
- 2 egg yolks
- 1 teaspoon ground coriander
- 1 teaspoon ground cumin
- 3 garlic cloves, minced
- 1 teaspoon dried oregano
- ½ teaspoon salt
- ½ teaspoon black pepper
- 1 lemon, juiced and zested
- ¼ cup fresh parsley, chopped
- ½ cup crumbled feta cheese
- Olive oil, for shaping
- Tzatziki, for dipping

Directions:
1. Combine all ingredients except olive oil in a large mixing bowl and mix until fully incorporated.
2. Form 12 meatballs, about 2 ounces each. Use olive oil on your hands so they don't stick to the meatballs. Set aside.
3. Select the Broil function on the COSORI Air Fryer Toaster Oven, set time to 12 minutes, then press Start/Cancel to preheat.
4. Place the meatballs on the food tray, then insert the tray at top position in the

preheated air fryer toaster oven. Press Start/Cancel.

5. Take out the meatballs when done and serve with a side of tzatziki.

- **Nutrition Info:** Calories: 129 kcal Total Fat: 6.4 g Saturated Fat: 0 g Cholesterol: 0 mg Sodium: 0 mg Total Carbs: 4.9 g Fiber: 0 g Sugar: 0 g Protein: 12.9 g

96. Sweet Potato Rosti

Servings: 2
Cooking Time: 15 Minutes
Ingredients:

- ½ lb. sweet potatoes, peeled, grated and squeezed
- 1 tablespoon fresh parsley, chopped finely
- Salt and ground black pepper, as required
- 2 tablespoons sour cream

Directions:

1. In a large bowl, mix together the grated sweet potato, parsley, salt, and black pepper.
2. Press "Power Button" of Air Fry Oven and turn the dial to select the "Air Fry" mode.
3. Press the Time button and again turn the dial to set the cooking time to 15 minutes.
4. Now push the Temp button and rotate the dial to set the temperature at 355 degrees F.
5. Press "Start/Pause" button to start.
6. When the unit beeps to show that it is preheated, open the lid and lightly, grease the sheet pan.
7. Arrange the sweet potato mixture into the "Sheet Pan" and shape it into an even circle.
8. Insert the "Sheet Pan" in the oven.
9. Cut the potato rosti into wedges.
10. Top with the sour cream and serve immediately.

- **Nutrition Info:** Calories: 160 Cal Total Fat: 2.7 g Saturated Fat: 1.6 g Cholesterol: 5 mg Sodium: 95 mg Total Carbs: 32.3 g Fiber: 4.7 g Sugar: 0.6 g Protein: 2.2 g

97. Turkey And Almonds

Servings: 2
Cooking Time: 10 Minutes
Ingredients:

- 1 big turkey breast, skinless; boneless and halved
- 2 shallots; chopped
- 1/3 cup almonds; chopped
- 1 tbsp. sweet paprika
- 2 tbsp. olive oil
- Salt and black pepper to taste.

Directions:

1. In a pan that fits the air fryer, combine the turkey with all the other ingredients, toss.
2. Put the pan in the machine and cook at 370°F for 25 minutes
3. Divide everything between plates and serve.

- **Nutrition Info:** Calories: 274; Fat: 12g; Fiber: 3g; Carbs: 5g; Protein: 14g

98. Carrot And Beef Cocktail Balls

Servings: 10
Cooking Time: 20 Minutes
Ingredients:

- 1-pound ground beef
- 2 carrots
- 1 red onion, peeled and chopped
- 2 cloves garlic
- 1/2 teaspoon dried rosemary, crushed
- 1/2 teaspoon dried basil
- 1 teaspoon dried oregano
- 1 egg
- 3/4 cup breadcrumbs
- 1/2 teaspoon salt
- 1/2 teaspoon black pepper, or to taste
- 1 cup plain flour

Directions:

1. Preparing the ingredients. Place ground beef in a large bowl.
2. In a food processor, pulse the carrot, onion and garlic; transfer the vegetable mixture to a large-sized bowl.
3. Then, add the rosemary, basil, oregano, egg, breadcrumbs, salt, and black pepper.
4. Shape the mixture into even balls; refrigerate for about 30 minutes.
5. Roll the balls into the flour.
6. Air frying. Close air fryer lid.
7. Then, air-fry the balls at 350 degrees f for about 20 minutes, turning occasionally; work with batches. Serve with toothpicks.

- **Nutrition Info:** Calories 284 Total fat 7.9 g Saturated fat 1.4 g Cholesterol 36 mg

Sodium 704 mg Total carbs 46 g Fiber 3.6 g
Sugar 5.5 g Protein 17.9 g

99. Herb-roasted Turkey Breast

Servings: 8
Cooking Time: 60 Minutes
Ingredients:

- 3 lb turkey breast
- Rub Ingredients:
- 2 tbsp olive oil
- 2 tbsp lemon juice
- 1 tbsp minced Garlic
- 2 tsp ground mustard
- 2 tsp kosher salt
- 1 tsp pepper
- 1 tsp dried rosemary
- 1 tsp dried thyme
- 1 tsp ground sage

Directions:

1. Take a small bowl and thoroughly combine the Rub Ingredients: in it. Rub this on the outside of the turkey breast and under any loose skin.
2. Place the coated turkey breast keeping skin side up on a cooking tray.
3. Place the drip pan at the bottom of the cooking chamber of the Instant Pot Duo Crisp Air Fryer. Select Air Fry option, post this, adjust the temperature to 360°F and the time to one hour, then touch start.
4. When preheated, add the food to the cooking tray in the lowest position. Close the lid for cooking.
5. When the Air Fry program is complete, check to make sure that the thickest portion of the meat reads at least 160°F, remove the turkey and let it rest for 10 minutes before slicing and serving.
- **Nutrition Info:** Calories 214, Total Fat 10g, Total Carbs 2g, Protein 29g

100. Fried Whole Chicken

Servings: 4
Cooking Time: 70 Minutes
Ingredients:

- 1 Whole chicken
- 2 Tbsp or spray of oil of choice
- 1 tsp garlic powder

- 1 tsp onion powder
- 1 tsp paprika
- 1 tsp Italian seasoning
- 2 Tbsp Montreal Steak Seasoning (or salt and pepper to taste)
- 1.5 cup chicken broth

Directions:

1. Truss and wash the chicken.
2. Mix the seasoning and rub a little amount on the chicken.
3. Pour the broth inside the Instant Pot Duo Crisp Air Fryer.
4. Place the chicken in the air fryer basket.
5. Select the option Air Fry and Close the Air Fryer lid and cook for 25 minutes.
6. Spray or rub the top of the chicken with oil and rub it with half of the seasoning.
7. Close the air fryer lid and air fry again at 400°F for 10 minutes.
8. Flip the chicken, spray it with oil, and rub with the remaining seasoning.
9. Again air fry it for another ten minutes.
10. Allow the chicken to rest for 10 minutes.
- **Nutrition Info:** Calories 436, Total Fat 28g, Total Carbs 4g, Protein 42g

101. Chicken Parmesan

Servings: 4
Cooking Time: 10 Minutes
Ingredients:

- 2 (6-oz.boneless, skinless chicken breasts
- 1 oz. pork rinds, crushed
- ½ cup grated Parmesan cheese, divided.
- 1 cup low-carb, no-sugar-added pasta sauce.
- 1 cup shredded mozzarella cheese, divided.
- 4 tbsp. full-fat mayonnaise, divided.
- ½ tsp. garlic powder.
- ¼ tsp. dried oregano.
- ½ tsp. dried parsley.

Directions:

1. Slice each chicken breast in half lengthwise and lb. out to 3/4-inch thickness. Sprinkle with garlic powder, oregano and parsley
2. Spread 1 tbsp. mayonnaise on top of each piece of chicken, then sprinkle ¼ cup mozzarella on each piece.

3. In a small bowl, mix the crushed pork rinds and Parmesan. Sprinkle the mixture on top of mozzarella

4. Pour sauce into 6-inch round baking pan and place chicken on top. Place pan into the air fryer basket. Adjust the temperature to 320 Degrees F and set the timer for 25 minutes

5. Cheese will be browned and internal temperature of the chicken will be at least 165 Degrees F when fully cooked. Serve warm.

- **Nutrition Info:** Calories: 393; Protein: 32g; Fiber: 1g; Fat: 28g; Carbs: 8g

102.Air Fryer Beef Steak

Servings: 4
Cooking Time: 15 Minutes
Ingredients:

- 1 tbsp. Olive oil
- Pepper and salt
- 2 pounds of ribeye steak

Directions:

1. Preparing the ingredients. Season meat on both sides with pepper and salt.
2. Rub all sides of meat with olive oil.
3. Preheat instant crisp air fryer to 356 degrees and spritz with olive oil.
4. Air frying. Close air fryer lid. Set temperature to 356°f, and set time to 7 minutes. Cook steak 7 minutes. Flip and cook an additional 6 minutes.
5. Let meat sit 2-5 minutes to rest. Slice and serve with salad.

- **Nutrition Info:** Calories: 233; Fat: 19g; Protein:16g; Sugar:0g

103.Maple Chicken Thighs

Servings: 4
Cooking Time: 30 Minutes
Ingredients:

- 4 large chicken thighs, bone-in
- 2 tablespoons French mustard
- 2 tablespoons Dijon mustard
- 1 clove minced garlic
- 1/2 teaspoon dried marjoram
- 2 tablespoons maple syrup

Directions:

1. Mix chicken with everything in a bowl and coat it well.
2. Place the chicken along with its marinade in the baking pan.
3. Press "Power Button" of Air Fry Oven and turn the dial to select the "Bake" mode.
4. Press the Time button and again turn the dial to set the cooking time to 30 minutes.
5. Now push the Temp button and rotate the dial to set the temperature at 370 degrees F.
6. Once preheated, place the baking pan inside and close its lid.
7. Serve warm.

- **Nutrition Info:** Calories 301 Total Fat 15.8 g Saturated Fat 2.7 g Cholesterol 75 mg Sodium 189 mg Total Carbs 31.7 g Fiber 0.3 g Sugar 0.1 g Protein 28.2 g

104.Easy Prosciutto Grilled Cheese

Servings: 1
Cooking Time: 5 Minutes
Ingredients:

- 2 slices muenster cheese
- 2 slices white bread
- Four thinly-shaved pieces of prosciutto
- 1 tablespoon sweet and spicy pickles

Directions:

1. Set toaster oven to the Toast setting.
2. Place one slice of cheese on each piece of bread.
3. Put prosciutto on one slice and pickles on the other.
4. Transfer to a baking sheet and toast for 4 minutes or until the cheese is melted.
5. Combine the sides, cut, and serve.

- **Nutrition Info:** Calories: 460, Sodium: 2180 mg, Dietary Fiber: 0 g, Total Fat: 25.2 g, Total Carbs: 11.9 g, Protein: 44.2 g.

105.Lemon Pepper Turkey

Servings: 6
Cooking Time: 45 Minutes
Ingredients:

- 3 lbs. turkey breast
- 2 tablespoons oil
- 1 tablespoon Worcestershire sauce
- 1 teaspoon lemon pepper
- 1/2 teaspoon salt

Directions:

1. Whisk everything in a bowl and coat the turkey liberally.
2. Place the turkey in the Air fryer basket.
3. Press "Power Button" of Air Fry Oven and turn the dial to select the "Air Fry" mode.
4. Press the Time button and again turn the dial to set the cooking time to 45 minutes.
5. Now push the Temp button and rotate the dial to set the temperature at 375 degrees F.
6. Once preheated, place the air fryer basket inside and close its lid.
7. Serve warm.

- **Nutrition Info:** Calories 391 Total Fat 2.8 g Saturated Fat 0.6 g Cholesterol 330 mg Sodium 62 mg Total Carbs 36.5 g Fiber 9.2 g Sugar 4.5 g Protein 6.6

106.Philly Cheesesteak Egg Rolls

Servings: 4-5
Cooking Time: 20 Minutes
Ingredients:

- 1 egg
- 1 tablespoon milk
- 2 tablespoons olive oil
- 1 small red onion
- 1 small red bell pepper
- 1 small green bell pepper
- 1 pound thinly slice roast beef
- 8 ounces shredded pepper jack cheese
- 8 ounces shredded provolone cheese
- 8-10 egg roll skins
- Salt and pepper

Directions:

1. Start by preheating toaster oven to 425°F.
2. Mix together egg and milk in a shallow bowl and set aside for later use.
3. Chop onions and bell peppers into small pieces.
4. Heat the oil in a medium sauce pan and add the onions and peppers.
5. Cook onions and peppers for 2–3 minutes until softened.
6. Add roast beef to the pan and sauté for another 5 minutes.
7. Add salt and pepper to taste.
8. Add cheese and mix together until melted.

9. Remove from heat and drain liquid from pan.
10. Roll the egg roll skins flat.
11. Add equal parts of the mix to each egg roll and roll them up per the instructions on the package.
12. Brush each egg roll with the egg mixture.
13. Line a pan with parchment paper and lay egg rolls seam-side down with a gap between each roll.
14. Bake for 20–25 minutes, depending on your preference of egg roll crispness.

- **Nutrition Info:** Calories: 769, Sodium: 1114 mg, Dietary Fiber: 2.1 g, Total Fat: 39.9 g, Total Carbs: 41.4 g, Protein: 58.4 g.

107.Cheese-stuffed Meatballs

Servings: 4
Cooking Time: 10 Minutes
Ingredients:

- ⅓ cup soft bread crumbs
- 3 tablespoons milk
- 1 tablespoon ketchup
- 1 egg
- ½ teaspoon dried marjoram
- Pinch salt
- Freshly ground black pepper
- 1-pound 95 percent lean ground beef
- 20 ½-inch cubes of cheese
- Olive oil for misting

Directions:

1. Preparing the ingredients. In a large bowl, combine the bread crumbs, milk, ketchup, egg, marjoram, salt, and pepper, and mix well. Add the ground beef and mix gently but thoroughly with your hands. Form the mixture into 20 meatballs. Shape each meatball around a cheese cube. Mist the meatballs with olive oil and put into the instant crisp air fryer basket.
2. Air frying. Close air fryer lid. Bake for 10 to 13 minutes or until the meatballs register 165°f on a meat thermometer.

- **Nutrition Info:** Calories: 393; Fat: 17g; Protein:50g; Fiber:0g

108.Crisp Chicken Casserole

Servings: 4

Cooking Time: 15 Minutes

Ingredients:

- 3 cup chicken, shredded
- 12 oz bag egg noodles
- 1/2 large onion
- 1/2 cup chopped carrots
- 1/4 cup frozen peas
- 1/4 cup frozen broccoli pieces
- 2 stalks celery chopped
- 5 cup chicken broth
- 1 tsp garlic powder
- salt and pepper to taste
- 1 cup cheddar cheese, shredded
- 1 package French's onions
- 1/4 cup sour cream
- 1 can cream of chicken and mushroom soup

Directions:

1. Place the chicken, vegetables, garlic powder, salt and pepper, and broth and stir. Then place it into the Instant Pot Duo Crisp Air Fryer Basket.
2. Press or lightly stir the egg noodles into the mix until damp/wet.
3. Select the option Air Fryer and cook for 4 minutes.
4. Stir in the sour cream, can of soup, cheese, and 1/3 of the French's onions.
5. Top with the remaining French's onions and close the Air Fryer lid and cook for about 10 more minutes.
- **Nutrition Info:** Calories 301, Total Fat 17g, Total Carbs 17g, Protein 20g

109.Pumpkin Pancakes

Servings: 4
Cooking Time: 12 Minutes

Ingredients:

- 1 square puff pastry
- 3 tablespoons pumpkin filling
- 1 small egg, beaten

Directions:

1. Roll out a square of puff pastry and layer it with pumpkin pie filling, leaving about ¼-inch space around the edges.
2. Cut it up into 8 equal sized square pieces and coat the edges with beaten egg.
3. Press "Power Button" of Air Fry Oven and turn the dial to select the "Air Fry" mode.

4. Press the Time button and again turn the dial to set the cooking time to 12 minutes.
5. Now push the Temp button and rotate the dial to set the temperature at 355 degrees F.
6. Press "Start/Pause" button to start.
7. When the unit beeps to show that it is preheated, open the lid.
8. Arrange the squares into a greased "Sheet Pan" and insert in the oven.
9. Serve warm.
- **Nutrition Info:** Calories: 109 Cal Total Fat: 6.7 g Saturated Fat: 1.8 g Cholesterol: 34 mg Sodium: 87 mg Total Carbs: 9.8 g Fiber: 0.5 g Sugar: 2.6 g Protein: 2.4 g

110.Creamy Green Beans And Tomatoes

Servings: 4
Cooking Time: 20 Minutes

Ingredients:

- 1 pound green beans, trimmed and halved
- ½ pound cherry tomatoes, halved
- 2 tablespoons olive oil
- 1 teaspoon oregano, dried
- 1 teaspoon basil, dried
- Salt and black pepper to the taste
- 1 cup heavy cream
- ½ tablespoon cilantro, chopped

Directions:

1. In your air fryer's pan, combine the green beans with the tomatoes and the other Ingredients:, toss and cook at 360 degrees F for 20 minutes.
2. Divide the mix between plates and serve.
- **Nutrition Info:** Calories 174, fat 5, fiber 7, carbs 11, protein 4

111.Tomato Frittata

Servings: 2
Cooking Time: 30 Minutes

Ingredients:

- 4 eggs
- ¼ cup onion, chopped
- ½ cup tomatoes, chopped
- ½ cup milk
- 1 cup Gouda cheese, shredded
- Salt, as required

Directions:

1. In a small baking pan, add all the ingredients and mix well.
2. Press "Power Button" of Air Fry Oven and turn the dial to select the "Air Fry" mode.
3. Press the Time button and again turn the dial to set the cooking time to 30 minutes.
4. Now push the Temp button and rotate the dial to set the temperature at 340 degrees F.
5. Press "Start/Pause" button to start.
6. When the unit beeps to show that it is preheated, open the lid.
7. Arrange the baking pan over the "Wire Rack" and insert in the oven.
8. Cut into 2 wedges and serve.
- **Nutrition Info:** Calories: 247 Cal Total Fat: 16.1 g Saturated Fat: 7.5 g Cholesterol: 332 mg Sodium: 417 mg Total Carbs: 7.30 g Fiber: 0.9 g Sugar: 5.2 g Protein: 18.6 g

112.Simple Lamb Bbq With Herbed Salt

Servings: 8
Cooking Time: 1 Hour 20 Minutes
Ingredients:
- 2 ½ tablespoons herb salt
- 2 tablespoons olive oil
- 4 pounds boneless leg of lamb, cut into 2-inch chunks

Directions:
1. Preheat the air fryer to 390 ºF.
2. Place the grill pan accessory in the air fryer.
3. Season the meat with the herb salt and brush with olive oil.
4. Grill the meat for 20 minutes per batch.
5. Make sure to flip the meat every 10 minutes for even cooking.
- **Nutrition Info:** Calories: 347 kcal Total Fat: 17.8 g Saturated Fat: 0 g Cholesterol: 0 mg Sodium: 0 mg Total Carbs: 0 g Fiber: 0 g Sugar: 0 g Protein: 46.6 g

113.Kale And Pine Nuts

Servings: 4
Cooking Time: 12 Minutes
Ingredients:
- 10 cups kale; torn
- 1/3 cup pine nuts
- 2 tbsp. lemon zest; grated
- 1 tbsp. lemon juice

- 2 tbsp. olive oil
- Salt and black pepper to taste.

Directions:
1. In a pan that fits the air fryer, combine all the ingredients, toss, introduce the pan in the machine and cook at 380°F for 15 minutes
2. Divide between plates and serve as a side dish.
- **Nutrition Info:** Calories: 121; Fat: 9g; Fiber: 2g; Carbs: 4g; Protein: 5g

114.Nutmeg Chicken Thighs

Servings: 4
Cooking Time: 10 Minutes
Ingredients:
- 2 lb. chicken thighs
- 2 tbsp. olive oil
- ½ tsp. nutmeg, ground
- A pinch of salt and black pepper

Directions:
1. Season the chicken thighs with salt and pepper and rub with the rest of the ingredients
2. Put the chicken thighs in air fryer's basket, cook at 360°F for 15 minutes on each side, divide between plates and serve.
- **Nutrition Info:** Calories: 271; Fat: 12g; Fiber: 4g; Carbs: 6g; Protein: 13g

115.Buttery Artichokes

Servings: 4
Cooking Time: 20 Minutes
Ingredients:
- 4 artichokes, trimmed and halved
- 3 garlic cloves, minced
- 1 tablespoon olive oil
- Salt and black pepper to the taste
- 4 tablespoons butter, melted
- ¼ teaspoon cumin, ground
- 1 tablespoon lemon zest, grated

Directions:
1. In a bowl, combine the artichokes with the oil, garlic and the other Ingredients:, toss well and transfer them to the air fryer's basket.

2. Cook for 20 minutes at 370 degrees F, divide between plates and serve as a side dish.
- **Nutrition Info:** Calories 214, fat 5, fiber 8, carbs 12, protein 5

116. Deviled Chicken

Servings: 8
Cooking Time: 40 Minutes
Ingredients:
- 2 tablespoons butter
- 2 cloves garlic, chopped
- 1 cup Dijon mustard
- 1/2 teaspoon cayenne pepper
- 1 1/2 cups panko breadcrumbs
- 3/4 cup Parmesan, freshly grated
- 1/4 cup chives, chopped
- 2 teaspoons paprika
- 8 small bone-in chicken thighs, skin removed

Directions:
1. Toss the chicken thighs with crumbs, cheese, chives, butter, and spices in a bowl and mix well to coat.
2. Transfer the chicken along with its spice mix to a baking pan.
3. Press "Power Button" of Air Fry Oven and turn the dial to select the "Air Fry" mode.
4. Press the Time button and again turn the dial to set the cooking time to 40 minutes.
5. Now push the Temp button and rotate the dial to set the temperature at 350 degrees F.
6. Once preheated, place the baking pan inside and close its lid.

7. Serve warm.
- **Nutrition Info:** Calories 380 Total Fat 20 g Saturated Fat 5 g Cholesterol 151 mg Sodium 686 mg Total Carbs 33 g Fiber 1 g Sugar 1.2 g Protein 21 g

117. Air Fryer Marinated Salmon

Servings: 4
Cooking Time: 12 Minutes
Ingredients:
- 4 salmon fillets or 1 1lb fillet cut into 4 pieces
- 1 Tbsp brown sugar
- ½ Tbsp Minced Garlic
- 6 Tbsps Soy Sauce
- ¼ cup Dijon Mustard
- 1 Green onions finely chopped

Directions:
1. Take a bowl and whisk together soy sauce, dijon mustard, brown sugar, and minced garlic. Pour this mixture over salmon fillets, making sure that all the fillets are covered. Refrigerate and marinate for 20-30 minutes.
2. Remove salmon fillets from marinade and place them in greased or lined on the tray in the Instant Pot Duo Crisp Air Fryer basket, close the lid.
3. Select the Air Fry option and Air Fry for around 12 minutes at 400°F.
4. Remove from Instant Pot Duo Crisp Air Fryer and top with chopped green onions.
- **Nutrition Info:** Calories 267, Total Fat 11g, Total Carbs 5g, Protein 37g

DINNER RECIPES

118.Chargrilled Halibut Niçoise With Vegetables

Servings: 6
Cooking Time: 15 Minutes
Ingredients:

- 1 ½ pounds halibut fillets
- Salt and pepper to taste
- 2 tablespoons olive oil
- 2 pounds mixed vegetables
- 4 cups torn lettuce leaves
- 1 cup cherry tomatoes, halved
- 4 large hard-boiled eggs, peeled and sliced

Directions:

1. Place the instant pot air fryer lid on and preheat the instant pot at 390 degrees F.
2. Place the grill pan accessory in the instant pot.
3. Rub the halibut with salt and pepper. Brush the fish with oil.
4. Place on the grill.
5. Surround the fish fillet with the mixed vegetables, close the air fryer lid and grill for 15 minutes.
6. Assemble the salad by serving the fish fillet with mixed grilled vegetables, lettuce, cherry tomatoes, and hard-boiled eggs.
- **Nutrition Info:** Calories: 312; Carbs:16.8 g; Protein: 19.8g; Fat: 18.3g

119.Red Hot Chili Fish Curry

Servings: 4
Cooking Time: 20 Minutes
Ingredients:

- 2 tablespoons sunflower oil
- 1 pound fish, chopped
- 2 red chilies, chopped
- 1 tablespoon coriander powder
- 1 teaspoon red curry paste
- 1 cup coconut milk
- Salt and white pepper, to taste
- 1/2 teaspoon fenugreek seeds
- 1 shallot, minced
- 1 garlic clove, minced
- 1 ripe tomato, pureed

Directions:

1. Preheat your Air Fryer to 380 degrees F; brush the cooking basket with 1 tablespoon of sunflower oil.
2. Cook your fish for 10 minutes on both sides. Transfer to the baking pan that is previously greased with the remaining tablespoon of sunflower oil.
3. Add the remaining ingredients and reduce the heat to 350 degrees F. Continue to cook an additional 10 to 12 minutes or until everything is heated through. Enjoy!
- **Nutrition Info:** 298 Calories; 18g Fat; 4g Carbs; 23g Protein; 7g Sugars; 7g Fiber

120.Korean Beef Bowl

Servings: 4
Cooking Time: 18 Minutes
Ingredients:

- 1 tablespoon minced garlic
- 1 teaspoon ground ginger
- 4 oz chive stems, chopped
- 2 tablespoon apple cider vinegar
- 1 teaspoon stevia extract
- 1 tablespoon flax seeds
- 1 teaspoon olive oil
- 1 teaspoon olive oil
- 1-pound ground beef
- 4 tablespoon chicken stock

Directions:

1. Sprinkle the ground beef with the apple cider vinegar and stir the meat with the help of the spoon.
2. After this, sprinkle the ground beef with the ground ginger, minced garlic, and olive oil.
3. Mix it up.
4. Preheat the air fryer to 370 F.
5. Put the ground beef in the air fryer basket tray and cook it for 8 minutes.
6. After this, stir the ground beef carefully and sprinkle with the chopped chives, flax seeds, olive oil, and chicken stock.
7. Mix the dish up and cook it for 10 minutes more.
8. When the time is over – stir the dish carefully.
9. Serve Korean beef bowl immediately.
10. Enjoy!

- **Nutrition Info:** calories 258, fat 10.1, fiber 1.2, carbs 4.2, protein 35.3

Sodium 485mg Calcium 10% DV Potassium 7% DV

121. Air Fryer Buffalo Mushroom Poppers

Servings: 8
Cooking Time: 50 Minutes
Ingredients:

- 1 pound fresh whole button mushrooms
- 1/2 teaspoon kosher salt
- 3 tablespoons 1/3-less-fat cream cheese,
- 1/4 cup all-purpose flour
- Softened 1 jalapeño chile, seeded and minced
- Cooking spray
- 1/4 teaspoon black pepper
- 1 cup panko breadcrumbs
- 2 large eggs, lightly beaten
- 1/4 cup buffalo-style hot sauce
- 2 tablespoons chopped fresh chives
- 1/2 cup low-fat buttermilk
- 1/2 cup plain fat-free yogurt
- 2 ounces blue cheese, crumbled (about 1/2 cup)
- 3 tablespoons apple cider vinegar

Directions:

1. Remove stems from mushroom caps, chop stems and set caps aside. Stir together chopped mushroom stems, cream cheese, jalapeño, salt, and pepper. Stuff about 1 teaspoon of the mixture into each mushroom cap, rounding the filling to form a smooth ball.
2. Place panko in a bowl, place flour in a second bowl, and eggs in a third Coat mushrooms in flour, dip in egg mixture, and dredge in panko, pressing to adhere. Spray mushrooms well with cooking spray.
3. Place half of the mushrooms in air fryer basket, and cook for 20 minutes at 350°F. Transfer cooked mushrooms to a large bowl. Drizzle buffalo sauce over mushrooms; toss to coat then sprinkle with chives.
4. Stir buttermilk, yogurt, blue cheese, and cider vinegar in a small bowl. Serve mushroom poppers with blue cheese sauce.

- **Nutrition Info:** Calories 133 Fat 4g Saturated fat 2g Unsaturated fat 2g Protein 7g Carbohydrate 16g Fiber 1g Sugars 3g

122. Veggie Stuffed Bell Peppers

Servings: 6
Cooking Time: 25 Minutes
Ingredients:

- 6 large bell peppers, tops and seeds removed
- 1 carrot, peeled and finely chopped
- 1 potato, peeled and finely chopped
- ½ cup fresh peas, shelled
- 1/3 cup cheddar cheese, grated
- 2 garlic cloves, minced
- Salt and black pepper, to taste

Directions:

1. Preheat the Air fryer to 350 °F and grease an Air fryer basket.
2. Mix vegetables, garlic, salt and black pepper in a bowl.
3. Stuff the vegetable mixture in each bell pepper and arrange in the Air fryer pan.
4. Cook for about 20 minutes and top with cheddar cheese.
5. Cook for about 5 more minutes and dish out to serve warm.

- **Nutrition Info:** Calories: 101, Fat: 2.5g, Carbohydrates: 17.1g, Sugar: 7.4g, Protein: 4.1g, Sodium: 51mg

123. Creamy Breaded Shrimp

Servings: 3
Cooking Time: 20 Minutes
Ingredients:

- ¼ cup all-purpose flour
- 1 cup panko breadcrumbs
- 1 pound shrimp, peeled and deveined
- ½ cup mayonnaise
- ¼ cup sweet chili sauce
- 1 tablespoon Sriracha sauce

Directions:

1. Preheat the Air fryer to 400-degree F and grease an Air fryer basket.
2. Place flour in a shallow bowl and mix the mayonnaise, chili sauce, and Sriracha sauce in another bowl.
3. Place the breadcrumbs in a third bowl.

4. Coat each shrimp with the flour, dip into mayonnaise mixture and finally, dredge in the breadcrumbs.
5. Arrange half of the coated shrimps into the Air fryer basket and cook for about 10 minutes.
6. Dish out the coated shrimps onto serving plates and repeat with the remaining mixture.
*   **Nutrition Info:** Calories: 540, Fat: 18.2g, Carbohydrates: 33.1g, Sugar: 10.6g, Protein: 36.8g, Sodium: 813mg

124.Pollock With Kalamata Olives And Capers

Servings: 3
Cooking Time: 20 Minutes
Ingredients:
*   2 tablespoons olive oil
*   1 red onion, sliced
*   2 cloves garlic, chopped
*   1 Florina pepper, deveined and minced
*   3 pollock fillets,skinless
*   2 ripe tomatoes, diced
*   12 Kalamata olives, pitted and chopped
*   2 tablespoons capers
*   1 teaspoon oregano
*   1 teaspoon rosemary
*   Sea salt, to taste
*   1/2 cup white wine

Directions:
1. Start by preheating your Air Fryer to 360 degrees F. Heat the oil in a baking pan. Once hot, sauté the onion, garlic, and pepper for 2 to 3 minutes or until fragrant.
2. Add the fish fillets to the baking pan. Top with the tomatoes, olives, and capers. Sprinkle with the oregano, rosemary, and salt. Pour in white wine and transfer to the cooking basket.
3. Turn the temperature to 395 degrees F and bake for 10 minutes. Taste for seasoning and serve on individual plates, garnished with some extra Mediterranean herbs if desired. Enjoy!
*   **Nutrition Info:** 480 Calories; 37g Fat; 9g Carbs; 49g Protein; 5g Sugars; 2g Fiber

125.Herbed Eggplant

Servings: 2
Cooking Time: 15 Minutes
Ingredients:
*   1 large eggplant, cubed
*   ½ teaspoon dried marjoram, crushed
*   ½ teaspoon dried oregano, crushed
*   ½ teaspoon dried thyme, crushed
*   ½ teaspoon garlic powder
*   Salt and black pepper, to taste
*   Olive oil cooking spray

Directions:
1. Preheat the Air fryer to 390 degree F and grease an Air fryer basket.
2. Mix herbs, garlic powder, salt, and black pepper in a bowl.
3. Spray the eggplant cubes with cooking spray and rub with the herb mixture.
4. Arrange the eggplant cubes in the Air fryer basket and cook for about 15 minutes, flipping twice in between.
5. Dish out onto serving plates and serve hot.
*   **Nutrition Info:** Calories: 62, Fat: 0.5g, Carbohydrates: 14.5g, Sugar: 7.1g, Protein: 2.4g, Sodium: 83mg

126.Creamy Lemon Turkey

Servings: 4
Cooking Time: 20 Minutes
Ingredients:
*   1/3 cup sour cream
*   2 cloves garlic, finely minced 1/3 tsp. lemon zest
*   2 small-sized turkey breasts, skinless and cubed 1/3 cup thickened cream
*   2 tablespoons lemon juice
*   1 tsp. fresh marjoram, chopped
*   Salt and freshly cracked mixed peppercorns, to taste 1/2 cup scallion, chopped
*   1/2 can tomatoes, diced
*   1½ tablespoons canola oil

Directions:
1. Firstly, pat dry the turkey breast. Mix the remaining items; marinate the turkey for 2 hours.
2. Set the air fryer to cook at 355 °F. Brush the turkey with a nonstick spray; cook for 23

minutes, turning once. Serve with naan and enjoy!

- **Nutrition Info:** 260 Calories; 15.3g Fat; 8.9g Carbs; 28.6g Protein; 1.9g Sugars

127.Venetian Liver

Servings: 6
Cooking Time: 15-30;
Ingredients:

- 500g veal liver
- 2 white onions
- 100g of water
- 2 tbsp vinegar
- Salt and pepper to taste

Directions:

1. Chop the onion and put it inside the pan with the water. Set the air fryer to 1800C and cook for 20 minutes.
2. Add the liver cut into small pieces and vinegar, close the lid, and cook for an additional 10 minutes.
3. Add salt and pepper.
- **Nutrition Info:** Calories 131, Fat 14.19 g, Carbohydrates 16.40 g, Sugars 5.15 g, Protein 25.39 g, Cholesterol 350.41 mg

128.Lamb Skewers

Servings: 4
Cooking Time: 20 Minutes
Ingredients:

- 2 lb. lamb meat; cubed
- 2 red bell peppers; cut into medium pieces
- ¼ cup olive oil
- 2 tbsp. lemon juice
- 1 tbsp. oregano; dried
- 1 tbsp. red vinegar
- 1 tbsp. garlic; minced
- ½ tsp. rosemary; dried
- A pinch of salt and black pepper

Directions:

1. Take a bowl and mix all the ingredients and toss them well.
2. Thread the lamb and bell peppers on skewers, place them in your air fryer's basket and cook at 380°F for 10 minutes on each side. Divide between plates and serve with a side salad

- **Nutrition Info:** Calories: 274; Fat: 12g; Fiber: 3g; Carbs: 6g; Protein: 16g

129.Cheese Zucchini Boats

Servings: 2
Cooking Time: 20 Minutes
Ingredients:

- 2 medium zucchinis
- ¼ cup full-fat ricotta cheese
- ¼ cup shredded mozzarella cheese
- ¼ cup low-carb, no-sugar-added pasta sauce.
- 2 tbsp. grated vegetarian Parmesan cheese
- 1 tbsp. avocado oil
- ¼ tsp. garlic powder.
- ½ tsp. dried parsley.
- ¼ tsp. dried oregano.

Directions:

1. Cut off 1-inch from the top and bottom of each zucchini.
2. Slice zucchini in half lengthwise and use a spoon to scoop out a bit of the inside, making room for filling. Brush with oil and spoon 2 tbsp. pasta sauce into each shell
3. Take a medium bowl, mix ricotta, mozzarella, oregano, garlic powder and parsley
4. Spoon the mixture into each zucchini shell. Place stuffed zucchini shells into the air fryer basket.
5. Adjust the temperature to 350 Degrees F and set the timer for 20 minutes.
6. To remove from the fryer basket, use tongs or a spatula and carefully lift out. Top with Parmesan. Serve immediately.
- **Nutrition Info:** Calories: 215; Protein: 15g; Fiber: 7g; Fat: 19g; Carbs: 3g

130.Asparagus Frittata

Servings: 4
Cooking Time: 10 Minutes
Ingredients:

- 6 eggs
- 3 mushrooms, sliced
- 10 asparagus, chopped 1/4 cup half and half
- 2 tsp butter, melted
- 1 cup mozzarella cheese, shredded 1 tsp pepper

- 1 tsp salt

Directions:
1. Toss mushrooms and asparagus with melted butter and add into the air fryer basket.
2. Cook mushrooms and asparagus at 350 F for 5 minutes. Shake basket twice.
3. Meanwhile, in a bowl, whisk together eggs, half and half, pepper, and salt.
4. Transfer cook mushrooms and asparagus into the air fryer baking dish.
5. Pour egg mixture over mushrooms and asparagus.
6. Place dish in the air fryer and cook at 350 F for 5 minutes or until eggs are set.
7. Slice and serve.
- **Nutrition Info:** Calories 211 Fat 13 g Carbohydrates 4 g Sugar 1 g Protein 16 g Cholesterol 272 mg

131.Roasted Garlic Zucchini Rolls

Servings: 4
Cooking Time: 20 Minutes
Ingredients:
- 2 medium zucchinis
- ½ cup full-fat ricotta cheese
- ¼ white onion; peeled. And diced
- 2 cups spinach; chopped
- ¼ cup heavy cream
- ½ cup sliced baby portobello mushrooms
- ¾ cup shredded mozzarella cheese, divided.
- 2 tbsp. unsalted butter.
- 2 tbsp. vegetable broth.
- ½ tsp. finely minced roasted garlic
- ¼ tsp. dried oregano.
- ⅛ tsp. xanthan gum.
- ¼ tsp. salt
- ½ tsp. garlic powder.

Directions:
1. Using a mandoline or sharp knife, slice zucchini into long strips lengthwise. Place strips between paper towels to absorb moisture. Set aside
2. In a medium saucepan over medium heat, melt butter. Add onion and sauté until fragrant. Add garlic and sauté 30 seconds.

3. Pour in heavy cream, broth and xanthan gum. Turn off heat and whisk mixture until it begins to thicken, about 3 minutes.
4. Take a medium bowl, add ricotta, salt, garlic powder and oregano and mix well. Fold in spinach, mushrooms and ½ cup mozzarella
5. Pour half of the sauce into a 6-inch round baking pan. To assemble the rolls, place two strips of zucchini on a work surface. Spoon 2 tbsp. of ricotta mixture onto the slices and roll up. Place seam side down on top of sauce. Repeat with remaining ingredients
6. Pour remaining sauce over the rolls and sprinkle with remaining mozzarella. Cover with foil and place into the air fryer basket. Adjust the temperature to 350 Degrees F and set the timer for 20 minutes. In the last 5 minutes, remove the foil to brown the cheese. Serve immediately.
- **Nutrition Info:** Calories: 245; Protein: 15g; Fiber: 8g; Fat: 19g; Carbs: 1g

132.Healthy Mama Meatloaf

Servings: 8
Cooking Time: 40 Minutes
Ingredients:
- 1 tablespoon olive oil
- 1 green bell pepper, diced
- 1/2 cup diced sweet onion
- 1/2 teaspoon minced garlic
- 1-lb. ground beef
- 1 cup whole wheat bread crumbs
- 2 large eggs
- 3/4 cup shredded carrot
- 3/4 cup shredded zucchini
- salt and ground black pepper to taste
- 1/4 cup ketchup, or to taste

Directions:
1. Thoroughly mix ground beef with egg, onion, garlic, crumbs, and all the ingredients in a bowl.
2. Grease a meatloaf pan with oil or butter and spread the minced beef in the pan.
3. Press "Power Button" of Air Fry Oven and turn the dial to select the "Bake" mode.
4. Press the Time button and again turn the dial to set the cooking time to 40 minutes.

5. Now push the Temp button and rotate the dial to set the temperature at 375 degrees F.
6. Once preheated, place the beef baking pan in the oven and close its lid.
7. Slice and serve.
- **Nutrition Info:** Calories: 322 Cal Total Fat: 11.8 g Saturated Fat: 2.2 g Cholesterol: 56 mg Sodium: 321 mg Total Carbs: 14.6 g Fiber: 4.4 g Sugar: 8 g Protein: 17.3 g

133.Cinnamon Pork Rinds

Servings: 2
Cooking Time: 20 Minutes
Ingredients:
- 2 oz. pork rinds
- ¼ cup powdered erythritol
- 2 tbsp. unsalted butter; melted.
- ½ tsp. ground cinnamon.

Directions:
1. Take a large bowl, toss pork rinds and butter. Sprinkle with cinnamon and erythritol, then toss to evenly coat.
2. Place pork rinds into the air fryer basket. Adjust the temperature to 400 Degrees F and set the timer for 5 minutes. Serve immediately.
- **Nutrition Info:** Calories: 264; Protein: 13g; Fiber: 4g; Fat: 28g; Carbs: 15g

134.Sweet Chicken Breast

Servings: 4
Cooking Time: 12 Minutes
Ingredients:
- 1-pound chicken breast, boneless, skinless
- 3 tablespoon Stevia extract
- 1 teaspoon ground white pepper
- ½ teaspoon paprika
- 1 teaspoon cayenne pepper
- 1 teaspoon lemongrass
- 1 teaspoon lemon zest
- 1 tablespoon apple cider vinegar
- 1 tablespoon butter

Directions:
1. Sprinkle the chicken breast with the apple cider vinegar.
2. After this, rub the chicken breast with the ground white pepper, paprika, cayenne pepper, lemongrass, and lemon zest.

3. Leave the chicken breast for 5 minutes to marinate.
4. After this, rub the chicken breast with the stevia extract and leave it for 5 minutes more.
5. Preheat the air fryer to 380 F.
6. Rub the prepared chicken breast with the butter and place it in the air fryer basket tray.
7. Cook the chicken breast for 12 minutes.
8. Turn the chicken breast into another side after 6 minutes of cooking.
9. Serve the dish hot!
10. Enjoy!
- **Nutrition Info:** calories 160, fat 5.9, fiber 0.4, carbs 1, protein 24.2

135.Amazing Bacon And Potato Platter

Servings: 4
Cooking Time: 40 Minutes
Ingredients:
- 4 potatoes, halved
- 6 garlic cloves, squashed
- 4 streaky cut rashers bacon
- 2 sprigs rosemary
- 1 tbsp olive oil

Directions:
1. Preheat your air fryer to 392 f. In a mixing bowl, mix garlic, bacon, potatoes and rosemary; toss in oil. Place the mixture in your air fryer's cooking basket and roast for 25-30 minutes. Serve and enjoy!
- **Nutrition Info:** Calories: 336 Cal Total Fat: 18.5 g Saturated Fat: 0 g Cholesterol: 82 mg Sodium: 876 mg Total Carbs: 69.9 g Fiber: 0 g Sugar: 0 g Protein: 0 g

136.Italian Shrimp Scampi

Servings: 4
Cooking Time: 20 Minutes
Ingredients:
- 2 egg whites
- 1/2 cup coconut flour
- 1 cup Parmigiano-Reggiano, grated
- 1/2 teaspoon celery seeds
- 1/2 teaspoon porcini powder
- 1/2 teaspoon onion powder
- 1 teaspoon garlic powder

- 1/2 teaspoon dried rosemary
- 1/2 teaspoon sea salt
- 1/2 teaspoon ground black pepper
- 1 ½ pounds shrimp, deveined

Directions:
1. Whisk the egg with coconut flour and Parmigiano-Reggiano. Add in seasonings and mix to combine well.
2. Dip your shrimp in the batter. Roll until they are covered on all sides.
3. Cook in the preheated Air Fryer at 390 degrees F for 5 to 7 minutes or until golden brown. Work in batches. Serve with lemon wedges if desired.
- **Nutrition Info:** 300 Calories; 13g Fat; 5g Carbs; 47g Protein; 8g Sugars; 2g Fiber

137.Roasted Lamb

Servings: 4
Cooking Time: 1 Hour 30 Minutes
Ingredients:
- 2½ pounds half lamb leg roast, slits carved
- 2 garlic cloves, sliced into smaller slithers
- 1 tablespoon dried rosemary
- 1 tablespoon olive oil
- Cracked Himalayan rock salt and cracked peppercorns, to taste

Directions:
1. Preheat the Air fryer to 400 degree F and grease an Air fryer basket.
2. Insert the garlic slithers in the slits and brush with rosemary, oil, salt, and black pepper.
3. Arrange the lamb in the Air fryer basket and cook for about 15 minutes.
4. Set the Air fryer to 350 degree F on the Roast mode and cook for 1 hour and 15 minutes.
5. Dish out the lamb chops and serve hot.
- **Nutrition Info:** Calories: 246, Fat: 7.4g, Carbohydrates: 9.4g, Sugar: 6.5g, Protein: 37.2g, Sodium: 353mg

138.Grilled Chicken Tikka Masala

Servings: 4
Cooking Time: 20 Minutes
Ingredients:
- 1 tsp. Tikka Masala 1 tsp. fine sea salt

- 2 heaping tsps. whole grain mustard
- 2 tsps. coriander, ground 2 tablespoon olive oil
- 2 large-sized chicken breasts, skinless and halved lengthwise
- 2 tsp.s onion powder
- 1½ tablespoons cider vinegar Basmati rice, steamed
- 1/3 tsp. red pepper flakes, crushed

Directions:
1. Preheat the air fryer to 335 °For 4 minutes.
2. Toss your chicken together with the other ingredients, minus basmati rice. Let it stand at least 3 hours.
3. Cook for 25 minutes in your air fryer; check for doneness because the time depending on the size of the piece of chicken.
4. Serve immediately over warm basmati rice. Enjoy!
- **Nutrition Info:** 319 Calories; 20.1g Fat; 1.9g Carbs; 30.5g Protein; 0.1g Sugars

139.Easy Air Fryed Roasted Asparagus

Servings: 4
Cooking Time: 10 Minutes
Ingredients:
- 1 bunch fresh asparagus
- 1 ½ tsp herbs de provence
- Fresh lemon wedge (optional)
- 1 tablespoon olive oil or cooking spray
- Salt and pepper to taste

Directions:
1. Wash asparagus and trim off hard ends
2. Drizzle asparagus with olive oil and add seasonings
3. Place asparagus in air fryer and cook on 36 ºF for 6 to 10 minutes
4. Drizzle squeezed lemon over roasted asparagus.
- **Nutrition Info:** Calories 46 protein 2g fat 3g net carbs 1g

140.Homemade Beef Stroganoff

Servings: 3
Cooking Time: 20 Minutes
Ingredients:
- 1 pound thin steak
- 4 tbsp butter

- 1 whole onion, chopped
- 1 cup sour cream
- 8 oz mushrooms, sliced
- 4 cups beef broth
- 16 oz egg noodles, cooked

Directions:
1. Preheat your Air Fryer to 400 F. Using a microwave proof bowl, melt butter in a microwave oven. In a mixing bowl, mix the melted butter, sliced mushrooms, cream, onion, and beef broth.
2. Pour the mixture over steak and set aside for 10 minutes. Place the marinated beef in your fryer's cooking basket, and cook for 10 minutes. Serve with cooked egg noodles and enjoy!
- **Nutrition Info:** 456 Calories; 37g Fat; 1g Carbs; 21g Protein; 5g Sugars; 6g Fiber

141.Air Fryer Roasted Broccoli

Servings: 4
Cooking Time: 10 Minutes
Ingredients:
- 1 tsp. herbes de provence seasoning (optional)
- 4 cups fresh broccoli
- 1 tablespoon olive oil
- Salt and pepper to taste

Directions:
1. Drizzle or spray broccoli with olive and sprinkle seasoning throughout
2. Spray air fryer basket with cooking oil, place broccoli and cook for 5-8 minutes on 36 ºF
3. Open air fryer and examine broccoli after 5 minutes because different fryer brands cook at different rates.
- **Nutrition Info:** Calories 61 Fat 4g protein 3g net carbs 4g

142.Broccoli Crust Pizza

Servings: 4
Cooking Time: 20 Minutes
Ingredients:
- 3 cups riced broccoli, steamed and drained well
- ½ cup shredded mozzarella cheese
- ½ cup grated vegetarian Parmesan cheese.

- 1 large egg.
- 3 tbsp. low-carb Alfredo sauce

Directions:
1. Take a large bowl, mix broccoli, egg and Parmesan.
2. Cut a piece of parchment to fit your air fryer basket. Press out the pizza mixture to fit on the parchment, working in two batches if necessary. Place into the air fryer basket. Adjust the temperature to 370 Degrees F and set the timer for 5 minutes.
3. When the timer beeps, the crust should be firm enough to flip. If not, add 2 additional minutes. Flip crust.
4. Top with Alfredo sauce and mozzarella. Return to the air fryer basket and cook an additional 7 minutes or until cheese is golden and bubbling. Serve warm.
- **Nutrition Info:** Calories: 136; Protein: 9g; Fiber: 3g; Fat: 6g; Carbs:7g

143.Zucchini Muffins

Servings: 8
Cooking Time: 20 Minutes
Ingredients:
- 6 eggs
- 4 drops stevia 1/4 cup Swerve
- 1/3 cup coconut oil, melted 1 cup zucchini, grated
- 3/4 cup coconut flour 1/4 tsp ground nutmeg 1 tsp ground cinnamon 1/2 tsp baking soda

Directions:
1. Preheat the air fryer to 325 F.
2. Add all ingredients except zucchini in a bowl and mix well.
3. Add zucchini and stir well.
4. Pour batter into the silicone muffin molds and place into the air fryer basket.
5. Cook muffins for 20 minutes.
6. Serve and enjoy.
- **Nutrition Info:** Calories 136 Fat 12 g Carbohydrates 1 g Sugar 0.6 g Protein 4 g Cholesterol 123 mg

144.Greek-style Monkfish With Vegetables

Servings: 2
Cooking Time: 20 Minutes

Ingredients:
- 2 teaspoons olive oil
- 1 cup celery, sliced
- 2 bell peppers, sliced
- 1 teaspoon dried thyme
- 1/2 teaspoon dried marjoram
- 1/2 teaspoon dried rosemary
- 2 monkfish fillets
- 1 tablespoon soy sauce
- 2 tablespoons lime juice
- Coarse salt and ground black pepper, to taste
- 1 teaspoon cayenne pepper
- 1/2 cup Kalamata olives, pitted and sliced

Directions:
1. In a nonstick skillet, heat the olive oil for 1 minute. Once hot, sauté the celery and peppers until tender, about 4 minutes. Sprinkle with thyme, marjoram, and rosemary and set aside.
2. Toss the fish fillets with the soy sauce, lime juice, salt, black pepper, and cayenne pepper. Place the fish fillets in a lightly greased cooking basket and bake at 390 degrees F for 8 minutes.
3. Turn them over, add the olives, and cook an additional 4 minutes. Serve with the sautéed vegetables on the side.
- **Nutrition Info:** 292 Calories; 11g Fat; 1g Carbs; 22g Protein; 9g Sugars; 6g Fiber

145.Sesame Mustard Greens

Servings: 4
Cooking Time: 11 Minutes
Ingredients:
- 2 garlic cloves, minced
- 1 pound mustard greens, torn
- 1 tablespoon olive oil
- ½ cup yellow onion, sliced
- Salt and black pepper to the taste
- 3 tablespoons veggie stock
- ¼ teaspoon dark sesame oil

Directions:
1. Heat up a pan that fits your air fryer with the oil over medium heat, add onions, stir and brown them for 5 minutes.

2. Add garlic, stock, greens, salt and pepper, stir, introduce in your air fryer and cook at 350 °F for 6 minutes.
3. Add sesame oil, toss to coat, divide among plates and serve.
- **Nutrition Info:** Calories: 173; Fat: 6g; Fiber: 2g; Carbs: 4g; Protein: 5g

146.Homemade Pork Ratatouille

Servings: 4
Cooking Time: 25 Minutes
Ingredients:
- 4 pork sausages
- For ratatouille
- 1 pepper, chopped
- 2 zucchinis, chopped
- 1 eggplant, chopped
- 1 medium red onion, chopped
- 1 tbsp olive oil
- 1-ounce butterbean, drained
- 15 oz tomatoes, chopped
- 2 sprigs fresh thyme
- 1 tbsp balsamic vinegar
- 2 garlic cloves, minced
- 1 red chili, chopped

Directions:
1. Preheat your air fryer to 392 f. Mix pepper, eggplant, oil, onion, zucchinis, and add to the cooking basket. Roast for 20 minutes. Set aside to cool. Reduce air fryer temperature to 356 f. In a saucepan, mix prepared vegetables and the remaining ratatouille ingredients, and bring to a boil over medium heat.
2. Let the mixture simmer for 10 minutes; season with salt and pepper. Add sausages to your air fryer's basket and cook for 10-15 minutes. Serve the sausages with ratatouille.
- **Nutrition Info:** Calories: 232.3 Cal Total Fat: 11.5 g Saturated Fat: 4.0 g Cholesterol: 58.2 mg Sodium: 611 mg Total Carbs: 9.2 g Fiber: 1.7 g Sugar: 4.4 g Protein: 23.1 g

147.Morning Ham And Cheese Sandwich

Servings: 4
Cooking Time: 15 Minutes
Ingredients:
- 8 slices whole wheat bread

- 4 slices lean pork ham
- 4 slices cheese
- 8 slices tomato

Directions:

1. Preheat your air fryer to 360 f. Lay four slices of bread on a flat surface. Spread the slices with cheese, tomato, turkey and ham. Cover with the remaining slices to form sandwiches. Add the sandwiches to the air fryer cooking basket and cook for 10 minutes.
- **Nutrition Info:** Calories: 361 Cal Total Fat: 16.7 g Saturated Fat: 0 g Cholesterol: 0 mg Sodium: 1320 mg Total Carbs: 32.5 g Fiber: 2.3 g Sugar: 5.13 g Protein: 19.3 g

148.Chinese-style Spicy And Herby Beef

Servings: 4
Cooking Time: 20 Minutes
Ingredients:

- 1 pound flank steak, cut into small pieces
- 1 teaspoon fresh sage leaves, minced
- 1/3 cup olive oil
- 3 teaspoons sesame oil
- 3 tablespoons Shaoxing wine
- 2 tablespoons tamari
- 1 teaspoon hot sauce
- 1/8 teaspoon xanthum gum
- 1 teaspoon seasoned salt
- 3 cloves garlic,minced
- 1 teaspoon fresh rosemary leaves, finely minced
- 1/2 teaspoon freshly cracked black pepper

Directions:

1. Warm the oil in a sauté pan over a moderate heat. Now, sauté the garlic until just tender and fragrant.
2. Now, add the remaining ingredients. Toss to coat well.
3. Then, roast for about 18 minutes at 345 degrees F. Check doneness and serve warm.
- **Nutrition Info:** 354 Calories; 24g Fat; 8g Carbs; 21g Protein; 3g Sugars; 3g Fiber

149.Cheddar Pork Meatballs

Servings: 4 To 6
Cooking Time: 25 Minutes
Ingredients:

- 1 lb ground pork
- 1 large onion, chopped
- ½ tsp maple syrup
- 2 tsp mustard
- ½ cup chopped basil leaves
- Salt and black pepper to taste
- 2 tbsp. grated cheddar cheese

Directions:

1. In a mixing bowl, add the ground pork, onion, maple syrup, mustard, basil leaves, salt, pepper, and cheddar cheese; mix well. Use your hands to form bite-size balls. Place in the fryer basket and cook at 400 f for 10 minutes.
2. Slide out the fryer basket and shake it to toss the meatballs. Cook further for 5 minutes. Remove them onto a wire rack and serve with zoodles and marinara sauce.
- **Nutrition Info:** Calories: 300 Cal Total Fat: 24 g Saturated Fat: 9 g Cholesterol: 70 mg Sodium: 860 mg Total Carbs: 3 g Fiber: 0 g Sugar: 0 g Protein: 16 g

150.Grandma's Meatballs With Spicy Sauce

Servings: 4
Cooking Time: 20 Minutes
Ingredients:

- 4 tablespoons pork rinds
- 1/3 cup green onion
- 1 pound beef sausage meat
- 3 garlic cloves, minced
- 1/3 teaspoon ground black pepper
- Sea salt, to taste
- For the sauce:
- 2 tablespoons Worcestershire sauce
- 1/3 yellow onion, minced
- Dash of Tabasco sauce
- 1/3 cup tomato paste
- 1 teaspoon cumin powder
- 1/2 tablespoon balsamic vinegar

Directions:

1. Knead all of the above ingredients until everything is well incorporated.
2. Roll into balls and cook in the preheated Air Fryer at 365 degrees for 13 minutes.

3. In the meantime, in a saucepan, cook the ingredients for the sauce until thoroughly warmed. Serve your meatballs with the tomato sauce and enjoy!
- **Nutrition Info:** 360 Calories; 23g Fat; 6g Carbs; 23g Protein; 4g Sugars; 2g Fiber

151.Easy Marinated London Broil

Servings: 4
Cooking Time: 20 Minutes
Ingredients:
- For the marinade:
- 2 tablespoons Worcestershire sauce
- 2 garlic cloves, minced
- 1 tablespoon oil
- 2 tablespoons rice vinegar
- London Broil:
- 2 pounds London broil
- 2 tablespoons tomato paste
- Sea salt and cracked black pepper, to taste
- 1 tablespoon mustard

Directions:
1. Combine all the marinade ingredients in a mixing bowl; add the London boil to the bowl. Cover and let it marinate for 3 hours.
2. Preheat the Air Fryer to 400 degrees F. Spritz the Air Fryer grill pan with cooking oil.
3. Grill the marinated London broil in the preheated Air Fryer for 18 minutes. Turn London broil over, top with the tomato paste, salt, black pepper, and mustard.
4. Continue to grill an additional 10 minutes. Serve immediately.
- **Nutrition Info:** 517 Calories; 21g Fat; 5g Carbs; 70g Protein; 4g Sugars; 7g Fiber

152.Crumbly Oat Meatloaf

Servings: 8
Cooking Time: 60 Minutes
Ingredients:
- 2 lbs. ground beef
- 1 cup of salsa
- 3/4 cup Quaker Oats
- 1/2 cup chopped onion
- 1 large egg, beaten
- 1 tablespoon Worcestershire sauce
- Salt and black pepper to taste

Directions:
1. Thoroughly mix ground beef with salsa, oats, onion, egg, and all the ingredients in a bowl.
2. Grease a meatloaf pan with oil or butter and spread the minced beef in the pan.
3. Press "Power Button" of Air Fry Oven and turn the dial to select the "Bake" mode.
4. Press the Time button and again turn the dial to set the cooking time to 60 minutes.
5. Now push the Temp button and rotate the dial to set the temperature at 350 degrees F.
6. Once preheated, place the beef baking pan in the oven and close its lid.
7. Slice and serve.
- **Nutrition Info:** Calories: 412 Cal Total Fat: 24.8 g Saturated Fat: 12.4 g Cholesterol: 3 mg Sodium: 132 mg Total Carbs: 43.8 g Fiber: 3.9 g Sugar: 2.5 g Protein: 18.9 g

153.Pepper Pork Chops

Servings: 2
Cooking Time: 6 Minutes
Ingredients:
- 2 pork chops
- 1 egg white
- ¾ cup xanthum gum
- ½ teaspoon sea salt
- ¼ teaspoon freshly ground black pepper
- 1 oil mister

Directions:
1. Preheat the Air fryer to 400 degree F and grease an Air fryer basket.
2. Whisk egg white with salt and black pepper in a bowl and dip the pork chops in it.
3. Cover the bowl and marinate for about 20 minutes.
4. Pour the xanthum gum over both sides of the chops and spray with oil mister.
5. Arrange the chops in the Air fryer basket and cook for about 6 minutes.
6. Dish out in a bowl and serve warm.
- **Nutrition Info:** Calories: 541, Fat: 34g, Carbohydrates: 3.4g, Sugar: 1g, Protein: 20.3g, Sodium: 547mg

154.Baked Egg And Veggies

Servings: 2

Cooking Time: 20 Minutes

Ingredients:

- 1 cup fresh spinach; chopped
- 1 small zucchini, sliced lengthwise and quartered
- 1 medium Roma tomato; diced
- ½ medium green bell pepper; seeded and diced
- 2 large eggs.
- 2 tbsp. salted butter
- ¼ tsp. garlic powder.
- ¼ tsp. onion powder.
- ½ tsp. dried basil
- ¼ tsp. dried oregano.

Directions:

1. Grease two (4-inchramekins with 1 tbsp. butter each.
2. Take a large bowl, toss zucchini, bell pepper, spinach and tomatoes. Divide the mixture in two and place half in each ramekin.
3. Crack an egg on top of each ramekin and sprinkle with onion powder, garlic powder, basil and oregano. Place into the air fryer basket. Adjust the temperature to 330 Degrees F and set the timer for 10 minutes. Serve immediately.
- **Nutrition Info:** Calories: 150; Protein: 3g; Fiber: 2g; Fat: 10g; Carbs: 6g

155.Grilled Tasty Scallops

Servings: 2
Cooking Time: 10 Minutes

Ingredients:

- 1 pound sea scallops, cleaned and patted dry
- Salt and pepper to taste
- 3 dried chilies
- 2 tablespoon dried thyme
- 1 tablespoon dried oregano

- 1 tablespoon ground coriander
- 1 tablespoon ground fennel
- 2 teaspoons chipotle pepper

Directions:

1. Place the instant pot air fryer lid on and preheat the instant pot at 390 degrees F.
2. Place the grill pan accessory in the instant pot.
3. Mix all ingredients in a bowl.
4. Dump the scallops on the grill pan, close the air fryer lid and cook for 10 minutes.
- **Nutrition Info:** Calories:291 ; Carbs: 20.7g; Protein: 48.6g; Fat: 2.5g

156.Creamy Tuna Cakes

Servings: 4
Cooking Time: 15 Minutes

Ingredients:

- 2: 6-ouncescans tuna, drained
- 1½ tablespoon almond flour
- 1½ tablespoons mayonnaise
- 1 tablespoon fresh lemon juice
- 1 teaspoon dried dill
- 1 teaspoon garlic powder
- ½ teaspoon onion powder
- Pinch of salt and ground black pepper

Directions:

1. Preheat the Air fryer to 400-degree F and grease an Air fryer basket.
2. Mix the tuna, mayonnaise, almond flour, lemon juice, dill, and spices in a large bowl.
3. Make 4 equal-sized patties from the mixture and arrange in the Air fryer basket.
4. Cook for about 10 minutes and flip the sides.
5. Cook for 5 more minutes and dish out the tuna cakes in serving plates to serve warm.
- **Nutrition Info:** Calories: 200, Fat: 10.1g, Carbohydrates: 2.9g, Sugar: 0.8g, Protein: 23.4g, Sodium: 122mg

MEAT RECIPES

157. Turkey Grandma's Easy To Cook Wontons

Servings: x
Cooking Time: x
Ingredients:
- 1 ½ cup all-purpose flour
- ½ tsp. salt
- 5 tbsp. water
- 2 cups minced turkey
- 2 tbsp. oil
- 2 tsp. ginger-garlic paste
- 2 tsp. soya sauce
- 2 tsp. vinegar

Directions:
1. Squeeze the dough and cover it with plastic wrap and set aside. Next, cook the ingredients for the filling and try to ensure that the turkey is covered well with the sauce. Roll the dough and place the filling in the center. Now, wrap the dough to cover the filling and pinch the edges together. Pre heat the Breville smart oven at 200° F for 5 minutes.
2. Place the wontons in the fry basket and close it. Let them cook at the same temperature for another 20 minutes. Recommended sides are chili sauce or ketchup.

158. Sweet Sticky Chicken Wings

Servings: 4
Cooking Time: 20 Minutes
Ingredients:
- 16 chicken wings
- ¼ cup butter
- ¼ cup honey
- ½ tbsp salt
- 4 garlic cloves, minced
- ¾ cup potato starch

Directions:
1. Preheat Breville on AirFry function to 370 F. Coat the wings with potato starch and place them in a greased baking dish. Press Start and cook for 5 minutes. Whisk the rest of the ingredients in a bowl. Pour the sauce

over the wings and cook for another 10 minutes. Serve warm.

159. Mustard Chicken Breasts

Servings: 4
Cooking Time: 20 Minutes
Ingredients:
- ¼ cup flour
- 1 lb chicken breasts, sliced
- 1 tbsp Worcestershire sauce
- ¼ cup onions, chopped
- 1 ½ cups brown sugar
- ¼ cup yellow mustard
- ¾ cup water
- ½ cup ketchup

Directions:
1. Preheat Breville on AirFry function to 360 F. In a bowl, mix sugar, water, ketchup, onions, mustard, Worcestershire sauce, salt, and pepper. Stir until the sugar dissolves.
2. Flour the chicken slices and then dip it in the mustard mixture. Let marinate for 10 minutes. Place the chicken in a greased baking dish and press Start. Cook for 15 minutes. Serve immediately.

160. Pheasant Marinade Cutlet

Servings: x
Cooking Time: x
Ingredients:
- 2 cups sliced pheasant
- 1 big capsicum (Cut this capsicum into big cubes)
- 1 onion (Cut it into quarters. Now separate the layers carefully.)
- 5 tbsp. gram flour
- A pinch of salt to taste
- For the filling:
- 2 cup fresh green coriander
- ½ cup mint leaves
- 4 tsp. fennel
- 2 tbsp. ginger-garlic paste
- 1 small onion
- 6-7 flakes garlic (optional)
- Salt to taste
- 3 tbsp. lemon juice

Directions:

1. You will first need to make the sauce. Add the ingredients to a blender and make a thick paste. Slit the pieces of pheasant and stuff half the paste into the cavity obtained. Take the remaining paste and add it to the gram flour and salt.
2. Toss the pieces of pheasant in this mixture and set aside. Apply a little bit of the mixture on the capsicum and onion. Place these on a stick along with the pheasant pieces. Pre heat the Breville smart oven at 290 Fahrenheit for around 5 minutes. Open the basket. Arrange the satay sticks properly. Close the basket.
3. Keep the sticks with the mutton at 180 degrees for around half an hour while the sticks with the vegetables are to be kept at the same temperature for only 7 minutes. Turn the sticks in between so that one side does not get burnt and also to provide a uniform cook.

161.Rosemary Chicken Breasts

Servings: 2
Cooking Time: 15minutes
Ingredients:

- 2 chicken breasts
- Salt and black pepper to taste
- ½ cup dried rosemary
- 1 tbsp butter, melted

Directions:

1. Preheat Cuisinart on Air Fry function to 390 F. Lay a foil on a flat surface. Place the breasts on the foil, sprinkle with rosemary, tarragon, salt, and pepper and and drizzle the butter.
2. Wrap the foil around the breasts. Place the wrapped chicken in the AirFryer basket and fit in the baking tray; cook for 12 minutes. Remove and carefully unwrap. Serve with the sauce extract and steamed veggies.

162.Herby Turkey Balls

Servings:2
Cooking Time: 20 Minutes
Ingredients:

- ½ lb ground turkey

- 1 egg, beaten
- 1 cup breadcrumbs
- 1 tbsp dried thyme
- ½ tbsp dried parsley
- Salt and black pepper to taste

Directions:

1. Preheat Breville on AirFry function to 350 F. In a bowl, place ground turkey, thyme, parsley, salt, and pepper. Mix well and shape the mixture into balls. Dip in breadcrumbs, then in the egg, and finally in the breadcrumbs again. Place the nuggets in the basket and cook for 15 minutes.

163.Tuscan Air Fried Veal Loin

Servings: 3 Veal Chops
Cooking Time: 12 Minutes
Ingredients:

- 1½ teaspoons crushed fennel seeds
- 1 tablespoon minced fresh rosemary leaves
- 1 tablespoon minced garlic
- 1½ teaspoons lemon zest
- 1½ teaspoons salt
- ½ teaspoon red pepper flakes
- 2 tablespoons olive oil
- 3 (10-ounce / 284-g) bone-in veal loin, about ½ inch thick

Directions:

1. Combine all the ingredients, except for the veal loin, in a large bowl. Stir to mix well.
2. Dunk the loin in the mixture and press to submerge. Wrap the bowl in plastic and refrigerate for at least an hour to marinate.
3. Arrange the veal loin in the basket.
4. Put the air fryer basket on the baking pan and slide into Rack Position 2, select Air Fry, set temperature to 400ºF (205ºC) and set time to 12 minutes.
5. Flip the veal halfway through.
6. When cooking is complete, the internal temperature of the veal should reach at least 145ºF (63ºC) for medium rare.
7. Serve immediately.

164.Sherry Grilled Chicken

Servings: 2
Cooking Time: 25 Minutes
Ingredients:

- 2 chicken breasts, cubed
- 2 garlic clove, minced
- ½ cup ketchup
- ½ tbsp ginger, minced
- ½ cup soy sauce
- 2 tbsp sherry
- ½ cup pineapple juice
- 2 tbsp apple cider vinegar
- ½ cup brown sugar

Directions:

1. In a bowl, mix ketchup, pineapple juice, sugar, cider vinegar, and ginger. Heat the mixture in a frying pan over low heat. Cover chicken with the soy sauce and sherry; pour the hot sauce on top. Set aside for 15 minutes to marinate.
2. Preheat your Cuisinart oven on Broil function to 360 F. Remove the chicken from the marinade, pat dry, and place it in the greased basket. Fit in a baking tray and cook for 15 minutes.

165.Olive Caper Chicken

Servings: 4
Cooking Time: 18 Minutes
Ingredients:

- 4 chicken breast, boneless and halves
- 12 olives, pitted and halved
- 2 cups cherry tomatoes
- 3 tbsp olive oil
- 3 tbsp capers, rinsed and drained
- Pepper
- Salt

Directions:

1. Fit the Cuisinart oven with the rack in position
2. In a bowl, toss tomatoes, capers, olives with 2 tablespoons of oil. Set aside.
3. Season chicken with pepper and salt.
4. Heat remaining oil in a pan over high heat.
5. Place chicken in the pan and cook for 4 minutes.
6. Transfer chicken in baking dish. Top with tomato mixture.
7. Set to bake at 450 F for 23 minutes. After 5 minutes place the baking dish in the preheated oven.
8. Serve and enjoy.

- **Nutrition Info:** Calories 251 Fat 15 g Carbohydrates 4.7 g Sugar 2.4 g Protein 24.8 g Cholesterol 72 mg

166.Lamb Pops

Servings:x
Cooking Time:x
Ingredients:

- 1 cup cubed lamb
- 1 ½ tsp. garlic paste
- Salt and pepper to taste
- 1 tsp. dry oregano
- 1 tsp. dry basil
- ½ cup hung curd
- 1 tsp. lemon juice
- 1 tsp. red chili flakes

Directions:

1. Add the ingredients into a separate bowl and mix them well to get a consistent mixture. Dip the lamb pieces in the above mixture and leave them aside for some time. Pre heat the Breville smart oven at 180° C for around 5 minutes.
2. Place the coated lamb pieces in the fry basket and close it properly. Let them cook at the same temperature for 20 more minutes.
3. Keep turning them over in the basket so that they are cooked properly. Serve with tomato ketchup.

167.Herb Beef Tips

Servings: 6
Cooking Time: 20 Minutes
Ingredients:

- 2 lbs sirloin steak, cut into 1-inch cubes
- 1/4 tsp red chili flakes
- 1/2 tsp pepper
- 1/2 tsp dried thyme
- 1 tsp onion powder
- 1 tsp dried oregano
- 2 tbsp lemon juice
- 2 tbsp water
- 1/4 cup olive oil
- 1 cup parsley, chopped
- 1 tsp garlic, minced
- 1/2 tsp salt

Directions:

1. Fit the Cuisinart oven with the rack in position
2. Add all ingredients into the zip-lock bag, seal bag shake well and place in the refrigerator for 1 hour.
3. Place marinated steak cubes into the parchment-lined baking pan.
4. Set to bake at 400 F for 25 minutes. After 5 minutes place the baking pan in the preheated oven.
5. Serve and enjoy.
- **Nutrition Info:** Calories 361 Fat 18 g Carbohydrates 1.6 g Sugar 0.4 g Protein 46.3 g Cholesterol 135 mg

168.Juicy Pork Ribs Ole

Servings: 4
Cooking Time: 25 Minutes
Ingredients:
- 1 rack of pork ribs
- 1/2 cup low-fat milk
- 1 tablespoon envelope taco seasoning mix
- 1 can tomato sauce
- 1/2 teaspoon ground black pepper
- 1 teaspoon seasoned salt
- 1 tablespoon cornstarch
- 1 teaspoon canola oil

Directions:
1. Preparing the Ingredients. Place all ingredients in a mixing dish; let them marinate for 1 hour.
2. Air Frying. Cook the marinated ribs approximately 25 minutes at 390 degrees F
3. Work with batches. Enjoy .

169.Fried Chicken Tenderloins

Servings: 4
Cooking Time: 15 Minutes
Ingredients:
- 8 chicken tenderloins
- 2 tbsp butter, softened
- 2 oz breadcrumbs
- 1 large egg, whisked

Directions:
1. Preheat Cuisinart on Air Fry function to 380 F. Combine butter and breadcrumbs in a bowl. Keep mixing and stirring until the mixture gets crumbly. Dip the chicken in the egg, then in the crumb mix. Place in the greased basket and fit in the baking tray; cook for 10 minutes, flipping once until crispy. Set on Broil function for crispier taste. Serve.

170.Kielbasa Sausage With Pineapple And Bell Peppers

Servings:2 To 4
Cooking Time: 10 Minutes
Ingredients:
- ¾ pound (340 g) kielbasa sausage, cut into ½-inch slices
- 1 (8-ounce / 227-g) can pineapple chunks in juice, drained
- 1 cup bell pepper chunks
- 1 tablespoon barbecue seasoning
- 1 tablespoon soy sauce
- Cooking spray

Directions:
1. Spritz the air fryer basket with cooking spray.
2. Combine all the ingredients in a large bowl. Toss to mix well.
3. Pour the sausage mixture in the basket.
4. Put the air fryer basket on the baking pan and slide into Rack Position 2, select Air Fry, set temperature to 390ºF (199ºC) and set time to 10 minutes.
5. After 5 minutes, remove from the oven. Stir the sausage mixture. Return to the oven and continue cooking.
6. When cooking is complete, the sausage should be lightly browned and the bell pepper and pineapple should be soft.
7. Serve immediately.

171.Sweet Pork Belly

Servings:6
Cooking Time: 35 Minutes
Ingredients:
- 2 pounds pork belly
- Salt and black pepper to taste
- 3 tbsp olive oil
- 3 tbsp honey

Directions:
1. Season the pork belly with salt and pepper. Grease a baking dish with olive oil. Add in

the meat and place in the oven. Select Bake function, adjust the temperature to 400 F, and press Start. Cook for 15 minutes. Brush with honey and cook for 10 more minutes. Serve with green salad.

172.Dijon Garlic Pork Tenderloin

Servings: 6
Cooking Time: 10 Minutes
Ingredients:

- 1 C. breadcrumbs
- Pinch of cayenne pepper
- 3 crushed garlic cloves
- 2 tbsp. ground ginger
- 2 tbsp. Dijon mustard
- 2 tbsp. raw honey
- 4 tbsp. water
- 2 tsp. salt
- 1 pound pork tenderloin, sliced into 1-inch rounds

Directions:

1. Preparing the Ingredients. With pepper and salt, season all sides of tenderloin.
2. Combine cayenne pepper, garlic, ginger, mustard, honey, and water until smooth.
3. Dip pork rounds into the honey mixture and then into breadcrumbs, ensuring they all get coated well.
4. Place coated pork rounds into your Cuisinart air fryer oven.
5. Air Frying. Set temperature to 400°F, and set time to 10 minutes. Cook 10 minutes at 400 degrees. Flip and then cook an additional 5 minutes until golden in color.
- **Nutrition Info:** CALORIES: 423; FAT: 18G; PROTEIN:31G; SUGAR:3G

173.Spicy Meatballs

Servings: 4
Cooking Time: 30 Minutes
Ingredients:

- 1 lb ground beef
- 4 oz cream cheese
- 1 tsp dried basil
- 2 tbsp Worcestershire sauce
- 1/3 cup milk
- 1/2 cup cheddar cheese, shredded
- 3/4 cup breadcrumbs

- 2 jalapenos, minced
- 1/2 onion, minced
- 1 tsp salt

Directions:

1. Fit the Cuisinart oven with the rack in position
2. Add all ingredients into the mixing bowl and mix until well combined.
3. Make small balls from the meat mixture and place it into the parchment-lined baking pan.
4. Set to bake at 400 F for 35 minutes. After 5 minutes place the baking pan in the preheated oven.
5. Serve and enjoy.
- **Nutrition Info:** Calories 472 Fat 23.2 g Carbohydrates 19.7 g Sugar 4.6 g Protein 43.7 g Cholesterol 149 mg

174.Juicy Spicy Lemon Kebab

Servings:x
Cooking Time:x
Ingredients:

- 2 tsp. garam masala
- 4 tbsp. chopped coriander
- 3 tbsp. cream
- 2 tbsp. coriander powder
- 4 tbsp. fresh mint (chopped)
- 3 tbsp. chopped capsicum
- 2 lb. chicken breasts cubed
- 3 onions chopped
- 5 green chilies-roughly chopped
- 1 ½ tbsp. ginger paste
- 1 ½ tsp. garlic paste
- 1 ½ tsp. salt
- 3 tsp. lemon juice
- 2 tbsp. peanut flour
- 3 eggs

Directions:

1. Mix the dry ingredients in a bowl. Make the mixture into a smooth paste and coat the chicken cubes with the mixture. Beat the eggs in a bowl and add a little salt to them. Dip the cubes in the egg mixture and coat them with sesame seeds and leave them in the refrigerator for an hour. Pre heat the Breville smart oven at 290 Fahrenheit for around 5 minutes.

2. Place the kebabs in the basket and let them cook for another 25 minutes at the same temperature. Turn the kebabs over in between the cooking process to get a uniform cook. Serve the kebabs with mint sauce.

175.Teriyaki Duck Legs

Servings: 6
Cooking Time: 2 Hours
Ingredients:
- 3 lbs. duck legs
- ½ cup teriyaki sauce
- 2 tbsp. soy sauce
- 2 tbsp. malt vinegar

Directions:
1. Place the rack in position 1 of the oven.
2. Place the duck legs, skin side up, in an 8x11-inch baking dish.
3. In a small bowl, whisk together remaining ingredients and pour around duck legs. Liquid needs to reach the skin level of duck, if not add water until it does.
4. Set the oven to convection bake on 300°F for 60 minutes. After 5 minutes, place the ducks in the oven and cook 90 minutes, or until tender.
5. Remove duck from the oven. Pour off cooking liquid into a small saucepan. Skim off fat and reserve. Bring sauce to a boil and cook until it reduces down, about 10 minutes, stirring occasionally.
6. Place the baking pan in position 2 of the oven. Place the duck legs in the fryer basket and brush with reserved fat and sauce. Place the basket in the oven and set to broil on 400°F for 10 minutes. Turn duck over halfway through and brush with fat and sauce again. Serve.
- **Nutrition Info:** Calories 608, Total Fat 20g, Saturated Fat 5g, Total Carbs 6g, Net Carbs 6g, Protein 101g, Sugar 5g, Fiber 0g, Sodium 1063mg, Potassium 111mg, Phosphorus 68mg

176.Pork Leg Roast With Candy Onions

Servings:4
Cooking Time: 52 Minutes

Ingredients:
- 2 teaspoons sesame oil
- 1 teaspoon dried sage, crushed
- 1 teaspoon cayenne pepper
- 1 rosemary sprig, chopped
- 1 thyme sprig, chopped
- Sea salt and ground black pepper, to taste
- 2 pounds (907 g) pork leg roast, scored
- ½ pound (227 g) candy onions, sliced
- 4 cloves garlic, finely chopped
- 2 chili peppers, minced

Directions:
1. In a mixing bowl, combine the sesame oil, sage, cayenne pepper, rosemary, thyme, salt and black pepper until well mixed. In another bowl, place the pork leg and brush with the seasoning mixture.
2. Place the seasoned pork leg in the baking pan. Put the baking pan into Rack Position 2, select Air Fry, set temperature to 400ºF (205ºC) and set time to 40 minutes.
3. After 20 minutes, remove from the oven. Flip the pork leg. Return the pan to the oven and continue cooking.
4. After another 20 minutes, add the candy onions, garlic, and chili peppers to the pan and air fry for another 12 minutes.
5. When cooking is complete, the pork leg should be browned.
6. Transfer the pork leg to a plate. Let cool for 5 minutes and slice. Spread the juices left in the pan over the pork and serve warm with the candy onions.

177.Simple & Healthy Baked Chicken Breasts

Servings: 6
Cooking Time: 20 Minutes
Ingredients:
- 6 chicken breasts, skinless & boneless
- 1/4 tsp paprika
- 1 tsp Italian seasoning
- 2 tbsp olive oil
- 1/4 tsp pepper
- 1/2 tsp seasoning salt

Directions:
1. Fit the Cuisinart oven with the rack in position

2. Brush chicken with oil and season with paprika, Italian seasoning, pepper, and salt.
3. Place chicken breasts into the baking dish.
4. Set to bake at 400 F for 25 minutes. After 5 minutes place the baking dish in the preheated oven.
5. Serve and enjoy.
- **Nutrition Info:** Calories 320 Fat 15.7 g Carbohydrates 0.2 g Sugar 0.1 g Protein 42.3 g Cholesterol 130 mg

178.Meatballs(16)

Servings: 6
Cooking Time: 12 Minutes
Ingredients:
- 1 egg
- 20 oz ground beef
- 1/2 cup parmesan cheese, grated
- 8 tbsp almond milk
- 6 garlic cloves, minced
- 3/4 cups almond meal
- 2 tbsp basil, chopped
- 2 tbsp parsley, chopped
- 1 tsp black pepper
- 1 tsp salt

Directions:
1. Fit the Cuisinart oven with the rack in position
2. Add all ingredients into the mixing bowl and mix until well combined.
3. Make small balls from the meat mixture and place it into the parchment-lined baking pan.
4. Set to bake at 350 F for 17 minutes. After 5 minutes place the baking pan in the preheated oven.
5. Serve and enjoy.
- **Nutrition Info:** Calories 331 Fat 19 g Carbohydrates 5.3 g Sugar 1.3 g Protein 35.3 g Cholesterol 117 mg

179.Pork Chops With Potatoes(1)

Servings: 4
Cooking Time: 35 Minutes
Ingredients:
- 4 pork chops, boneless
- 1/4 tsp ground oregano
- 1 tsp dried parsley

- 3 tbsp olive oil
- 1 oz ranch seasoning
- 2 1lbs potatoes, cut into bite-size pieces
- 1/4 tsp pepper
- Salt

Directions:
1. Fit the Cuisinart oven with the rack in position
2. Season pork chops with ranch seasoning and pepper.
3. Place pork chops into the center of the baking pan.
4. In a bowl, toss potatoes with oil, parsley, oregano, and salt.
5. Place potatoes around the pork chops.
6. Set to bake at 400 F for 40 minutes. After 5 minutes place the baking pan in the preheated oven.
7. Serve and enjoy.
- **Nutrition Info:** Calories 433 Fat 30.5 g Carbohydrates 15.4 g Sugar 0.6 g Protein 19.8 g Cholesterol 69 mg

180.Sriracha Beef And Broccoli

Servings:4
Cooking Time: 15 Minutes
Ingredients:
- 12 ounces (340 g) broccoli, cut into florets (about 4 cups)
- 1 pound (454 g) flat iron steak, cut into thin strips
- ½ teaspoon kosher salt
- ¾ cup soy sauce
- 1 teaspoon Sriracha sauce
- 3 tablespoons freshly squeezed orange juice
- 1 teaspoon cornstarch
- 1 medium onion, thinly sliced

Directions:
1. Line the baking pan with aluminum foil. Place the broccoli on top and sprinkle with 3 tablespoons of water. Seal the broccoli in the foil in a single layer.
2. Slide the baking pan into Rack Position 2, select Roast, set temperature to 375ºF (190ºC), and set time to 6 minutes.
3. While the broccoli steams, sprinkle the steak with the salt. In a small bowl, whisk together the soy sauce, Sriracha, orange

juice, and cornstarch. Place the onion and beef in a large bowl.

4. When cooking is complete, remove from the oven. Open the packet of broccoli and use tongs to transfer the broccoli to the bowl with the beef and onion, discarding the foil and remaining water. Pour the sauce over the beef and vegetables and toss to coat. Place the mixture in the baking pan.

5. Select Roast, set temperature to 375ºF (190ºC), and set time to 9 minutes.

6. After about 4 minutes, remove from the oven and gently toss the ingredients. Return to the oven and continue cooking.

7. When cooking is complete, the sauce should be thickened, the vegetables tender, and the beef barely pink in the center. Serve warm.

181. Garlic Venison With Red Chili Flakes

Servings:x
Cooking Time:x
Ingredients:
- 1 lb. boneless venison cut into Oregano Fingers
- 2 cup dry breadcrumbs
- 6 tbsp. corn flour
- 4 eggs
- 2 tsp. oregano
- 2 tsp. red chili flakes
- 2 tsp. garlic paste
- 1 ½ tbsp. ginger-garlic paste
- 4 tbsp. lemon juice
- 2 tsp. salt
- 1 tsp. red chili powder

Directions:
1. Mix all the ingredients for the marinade and put the venison Oregano Fingers inside and let it rest overnight.

2. Mix the breadcrumbs, oregano and red chili flakes well and place the marinated Oregano Fingers on this mixture. Cover it with plastic wrap and leave it till right before you serve to cook.

3. Pre heat the Breville smart oven at 160 degrees Fahrenheit for 5 minutes. Place the Oregano Fingers in the fry basket and close it. Let them cook at the same temperature for another 15 minutes or so. Toss the

Oregano Fingers well so that they are cooked uniformly. Drizzle the garlic paste and serve.

182. Pork Fried Rice With Scrambled Egg

Servings:4
Cooking Time: 12 Minutes
Ingredients:
- 3 scallions, diced (about ½ cup)
- ½ red bell pepper, diced (about ½ cup)
- 2 teaspoons sesame oil
- ½ pound (227 g) pork tenderloin, diced
- ½ cup frozen peas, thawed
- ½ cup roasted mushrooms
- ½ cup soy sauce
- 2 cups cooked rice
- 1 egg, beaten

Directions:
1. Place the scallions and red pepper in the baking pan. Drizzle with the sesame oil and toss the vegetables to coat them in the oil.

2. Slide the baking pan into Rack Position 2, select Roast, set temperature to 375ºF (190ºC), and set time to 12 minutes.

3. While the vegetables are cooking, place the pork in a large bowl. Add the peas, mushrooms, soy sauce, and rice and toss to coat the ingredients with the sauce.

4. After about 4 minutes, remove from the oven. Place the pork mixture on the pan and stir the scallions and peppers into the pork and rice. Return the pan to the oven and continue cooking.

5. After another 6 minutes, remove from the oven. Move the rice mixture to the sides to create an empty circle in the middle of the pan. Pour the egg in the circle. Return the pan to the oven and continue cooking.

6. When cooking is complete, remove from the oven and stir the egg to scramble it. Stir the egg into the fried rice mixture. Serve immediately.

183. Swiss Cheese Ham Muffins

Servings: 8
Cooking Time: 25 Minutes
Ingredients:
- 4 whole eggs, beaten

- 3 oz ham
- 1 cup milk
- 1 ½ cups Swiss cheese, grated
- Salt and black pepper to taste
- ¼ cup green onion, chopped

Directions:

1. Preheat your Cuisinart to 350 F on Air Fry. In a bowl, mix eggs, onion, salt, cheese, pepper, and milk. Prepare baking forms and place ham slices in each one. Top with the egg mixture.
2. Place the muffin forms in the baking tray and cook for 15 minutes. Let cool for 10 minutes. Serve.

184.Cripsy Crusted Pork Chops

Servings: 4
Cooking Time: 40 Minutes
Ingredients:

- 4 pork chops, boneless
- 1 cup parmesan cheese
- 1 tbsp olive oil
- 1 tsp garlic powder
- 1 cup breadcrumbs
- 1/2 tsp Italian seasoning
- Pepper
- Salt

Directions:

1. Fit the Cuisinart oven with the rack in position
2. In a shallow dish, mix breadcrumbs, parmesan cheese, Italian seasoning, garlic powder, pepper, and salt.
3. Brush pork chops with oil and coat with breadcrumb mixture.
4. Place coated pork chops in a baking pan.
5. Set to bake at 350 F for 45 minutes. After 5 minutes place the baking pan in the preheated oven.
6. Serve and enjoy.
- **Nutrition Info:** Calories 469 Fat 29.8 g Carbohydrates 20.8 g Sugar 1.9 g Protein 28.9 g Cholesterol 85 mg

185.Chili Pork Chops With Tomatoes & Rice

Servings: 4
Cooking Time: 40 Minutes + Marinating Time

Ingredients:

- 4 pork chops
- 1 lime juice
- Salt and black pepper to taste
- 1 tsp garlic powder
- 1 ½ cups white rice, cooked
- 2 tbsp olive oil
- 1 can (14.5 oz) tomato sauce
- 1 onion, chopped
- 3 garlic cloves, minced
- ½ tsp oregano
- 1 tsp chipotle chili

Directions:

1. Season pork with salt, pepper, and garlic powder. In a bowl, mix onion, garlic, chipotle, oregano, and tomato sauce. Add in the pork. Let sit for 1 hour. Then remove from the mixture and place in the basket. Fit in the baking tray and cook for 25 minutes on Air Fry at 350 F. Serve with rice.

186.Chicken Oregano Fingers

Servings:x
Cooking Time:x
Ingredients:

- 1 lb. boneless chicken breast cut into Oregano Fingers
- 2 cup dry breadcrumbs
- 2 tsp. oregano
- 1 ½ tbsp. ginger-garlic paste
- 4 tbsp. lemon juice
- 2 tsp. salt
- 1 tsp. pepper powder
- 1 tsp. red chili powder
- 6 tbsp. corn flour
- 4 eggs

Directions:

1. Mix all the ingredients for the marinade and put the chicken Oregano Fingers inside and let it rest overnight.
2. Mix the breadcrumbs, oregano and red chili flakes well and place the marinated Oregano Fingers on this mixture. Cover it with plastic wrap and leave it till right before you serve to cook.
3. Pre heat the Breville smart oven at 160 degrees Fahrenheit for 5 minutes. Place the Oregano Fingers in the fry basket and close

it. Let them cook at the same temperature for another 15 minutes or so. Toss the Oregano Fingers well so that they are cooked uniformly.

187.Spanish Chicken And Pepper Baguette

Servings:2
Cooking Time: 20 Minutes
Ingredients:
- 1¼ pounds (567 g) assorted small chicken parts, breasts cut into halves
- ¼ teaspoon salt
- ¼ teaspoon ground black pepper
- 2 teaspoons olive oil
- ½ pound (227 g) mini sweet peppers
- ¼ cup light mayonnaise
- ¼ teaspoon smoked paprika
- ½ clove garlic, crushed
- Baguette, for serving
- Cooking spray

Directions:
1. Spritz the air fryer basket with cooking spray.
2. Toss the chicken with salt, ground black pepper, and olive oil in a large bowl.
3. Arrange the sweet peppers and chicken in the basket.
4. Put the air fryer basket on the baking pan and slide into Rack Position 2, select Air Fry, set temperature to 375ºF (190ºC) and set time to 20 minutes.
5. Flip the chicken and transfer the peppers on a plate halfway through.
6. When cooking is complete, the chicken should be well browned.
7. Meanwhile, combine the mayo, paprika, and garlic in a small bowl. Stir to mix well.
8. Assemble the baguette with chicken and sweet pepper, then spread with mayo mixture and serve.

188.Ginger Chicken Wings

Servings: 3
Cooking Time: 25 Minutes
Ingredients:
- 1 pound chicken wings
- 1 tbsp cilantro
- Salt and black pepper to taste

- 1 garlic clove, minced
- 1 tbsp yogurt
- 2 tbsp honey
- ½ tbsp vinegar
- ½ tbsp ginger, minced

Directions:
1. Preheat Cuisinart on Air Fry to 360 F. Season wings with salt and pepper, place them in the basket and fit in the baking tray. Cook for 15 minutes, shaking once. In a bowl, mix the remaining ingredients. Top the chicken with sauce and cook for 5 more minutes. Serve.

189.Duck Breasts With Marmalade Balsamic Glaze

Servings:4
Cooking Time: 13 Minutes
Ingredients:
- 4 (6-ounce / 170-g) skin-on duck breasts
- 1 teaspoon salt
- ¼ cup orange marmalade
- 1 tablespoon white balsamic vinegar
- ¾ teaspoon ground black pepper

Directions:
1. Cut 10 slits into the skin of the duck breasts, then sprinkle with salt on both sides.
2. Place the breasts in the air fryer basket, skin side up.
3. Put the air fryer basket on the baking pan and slide into Rack Position 2, select Air Fry, set temperature to 400ºF (205ºC) and set time to 10 minutes.
4. Meanwhile, combine the remaining ingredients in a small bowl. Stir to mix well.
5. When cooking is complete, brush the duck skin with the marmalade mixture. Flip the breast and air fry for 3 more minutes or until the skin is crispy and the breast is well browned.
6. Serve immediately.

190.Tasty Steak Tips

Servings: 4
Cooking Time: 5 Minutes
Ingredients:
- 1 lb steak, cut into cubes
- 1 tsp olive oil

- 1/4 tsp garlic powder
- 1 tsp Montreal steak seasoning
- Pepper
- Salt

Directions:

1. Fit the Cuisinart oven with the rack in position 2.
2. In a bowl, add steak cubes and remaining ingredients and toss well.
3. Add marinated steak cubes to the air fryer basket then place an air fryer basket in the baking pan.
4. Place a baking pan on the oven rack. Set to air fry at 400 F for 5 minutes.
5. Serve and enjoy.
- **Nutrition Info:** Calories 236 Fat 6.8 g Carbohydrates 0.2 g Sugar 0 g Protein 41 g Cholesterol 102 mg

191.Italian Sausage Jambalaya

Servings:x
Cooking Time:x
Ingredients:

- 2 cups water
- 3 spicy Italian sausages
- 2 Tbsp extra-virgin olive oil
- 2 cups frozen mirepoix
- 1 cup canned crushed tomatoes
- 1½ tsp Cajun seasoning
- 2 (8.8-oz) packages precooked rice
- Salt and freshly ground black pepper, to taste

Directions:

1. Remove the casings from the sausage and discard, then crumble the meat.
2. In Breville smart oven over medium heat, heat the olive oil.
3. Brown the sausage, stirring occasionally, for about 3 minutes.
4. Add the mirepoix and cook until tender, about 4 minutes.
5. Stir in the tomatoes, Cajun seasoning, and rice. Season with salt and pepper.
6. Simmer for about 5 minutes, and serve.

192.Mustardy Chicken

Servings: 4
Cooking Time: 20 Minutes

Ingredients:

- 1 tsp garlic powder
- 4 chicken breasts, sliced
- 1 tbsp fresh thyme, chopped
- ½ cup dry white wine
- Salt and black pepper to taste
- ½ cup Dijon mustard
- 2 cups breadcrumbs
- 1 tbsp lemon zest
- 2 tbsp olive oil

Directions:

1. In a bowl, mix garlic, breadcrumbs, olive oil, lemon zest, salt, and pepper. In another bowl, mix mustard and wine.
2. Dip the chicken slices in the wine mixture and then coat in the crumb mixture. Place the prepared chicken in the greased basket and fit in the baking tray; cook for 15 minutes at 350 F on Air Fry function, shaking once until golden brown. Serve.

193.Lime-chili Chicken Wings

Servings: 2
Cooking Time: 25 Minutes
Ingredients:

- 9 chicken wings
- 2 tbsp hot chili sauce
- ½ tbsp lime juice
- ½ tbsp honey
- ½ tbsp kosher salt
- ½ tbsp black pepper

Directions:

1. Preheat Cuisinart on Air Fry function to 350 F. Mix the lime juice, honey, and chili sauce. Toss the mixture over the chicken wings. Put the chicken wings in the basket and fit in the baking tray; cook for 25 minutes. Shake every 5 minutes. Serve.

194.Quail Chili

Servings:x
Cooking Time:x
Ingredients:

- 1 lb. quail (Cut into cubes)
- 2 ½ tsp. ginger-garlic paste
- 1 tsp. red chili sauce
- 2 tbsp. tomato ketchup
- 2 tsp. soya sauce

- 1-2 tbsp. honey
- ¼ tsp. Ajinomoto
- ¼ tsp. salt
- ¼ tsp. red chili powder/black pepper
- A few drops of edible orange food coloring
- 2 tbsp. olive oil
- 1 ½ tsp. ginger garlic paste
- ½ tbsp. red chili sauce
- 1-2 tsp. red chili flakes

Directions:

1. Mix all the ingredients for the marinade and put the quail cubes inside and let it rest overnight.
2. Mix the breadcrumbs, oregano and red chili flakes well and place the marinated Oregano Fingers on this mixture. Cover it with plastic wrap and leave it till right before you serve to cook.
3. Pre heat the Breville smart oven at 160 degrees Fahrenheit for 5 minutes. Place the Oregano Fingers in the fry basket and close it. Let them cook at the same temperature for another 15 minutes or so. Toss the Oregano Fingers well so that they are cooked uniformly.

195.Pork Spicy Lemon Kebab

Servings:x
Cooking Time:x
Ingredients:

- 1 lb. boneless pork cubed
- 3 onions chopped
- 5 green chilies-roughly chopped
- 1 ½ tbsp. ginger paste
- 4 tbsp. fresh mint chopped
- 3 tbsp. chopped capsicum
- 3 eggs
- 2 ½ tbsp. white sesame seeds
- 1 ½ tsp. garlic paste
- 1 ½ tsp. salt
- 3 tsp. lemon juice
- 2 tsp. garam masala
- 4 tbsp. chopped coriander
- 3 tbsp. cream
- 2 tbsp. coriander powder

Directions:

1. Mix the dry ingredients in a bowl. Make the mixture into a smooth paste and coat the pork cubes with the mixture. Beat the eggs in a bowl and add a little salt to them. Dip the cubes in the egg mixture and coat them with sesame seeds and leave them in the refrigerator for an hour. Pre heat the Breville smart oven at 290 Fahrenheit for around 5 minutes.
2. Place the kebabs in the basket and let them cook for another 25 minutes at the same temperature. Turn the kebabs over in between the cooking process to get a uniform cook. Serve the kebabs with mint sauce.

FISH & SEAFOOD RECIPES

196.Pecan-crusted Catfish Fillets

Servings:4
Cooking Time: 12 Minutes
Ingredients:
- ½ cup pecan meal
- 1 teaspoon fine sea salt
- ¼ teaspoon ground black pepper
- 4 (4-ounce / 113-g) catfish fillets
- Avocado oil spray
- For Garnish (Optional):
- Fresh oregano
- Pecan halves

Directions:
1. Spray the air fryer basket with avocado oil spray.
2. Combine the pecan meal, sea salt, and black pepper in a large bowl. Dredge each catfish fillet in the meal mixture, turning until well coated. Spritz the fillets with avocado oil spray, then transfer to the basket.
3. Put the air fryer basket on the baking pan and slide into Rack Position 2, select Air Fry, set temperature to 375ºF (190ºC), and set time to 12 minutes.
4. Flip the fillets halfway through the cooking time.
5. When cooking is complete, the fish should be cooked through and no longer translucent. Remove from the oven and sprinkle the oregano sprigs and pecan halves on top for garnish, if desired. Serve immediately.

197.Lemon Tilapia

Servings:4
Cooking Time: 12 Minutes
Ingredients:
- 1 tablespoon olive oil
- 1 tablespoon lemon juice
- 1 teaspoon minced garlic
- ½ teaspoon chili powder
- 4 tilapia fillets

Directions:
1. Line the baking pan with parchment paper.
2. In a shallow bowl, stir together the olive oil, lemon juice, garlic, and chili powder to

make a marinade. Put the tilapia fillets in the bowl, turning to coat evenly.
3. Place the fillets in the baking pan in a single layer.
4. Put the air fryer basket on the baking pan and slide into Rack Position 2, select Air Fry, set temperature to 375ºF (190ºC), and set time to 12 minutes.
5. When cooked, the fish will flake apart with a fork. Remove from the oven to a plate and serve hot.

198.Breaded Seafood

Servings:4
Cooking Time: 15 Minutes
Ingredients:
- 1 lb scallops, mussels, fish fillets, prawns, shrimp
- 2 eggs, lightly beaten
- Salt and black pepper to taste
- 1 cup breadcrumbs mixed with zest of 1 lemon

Directions:
1. Dip the seafood pieces into the eggs and season with salt and black pepper. Coat in the crumbs and spray with cooking spray. Arrange them on the frying basket and press Start. Cook for 10 minutes at 400 F on AirFry function. Serve with lemon wedges.

199.Easy Scallops

Servings:2
Cooking Time: 4 Minutes
Ingredients:
- 12 medium sea scallops, rinsed and patted dry
- 1 teaspoon fine sea salt
- ¾ teaspoon ground black pepper, plus more for garnish
- Fresh thyme leaves, for garnish (optional)
- Avocado oil spray

Directions:
1. Coat the air fryer basket with avocado oil spray.
2. Place the scallops in a medium bowl and spritz with avocado oil spray. Sprinkle the salt and pepper to season.

3. Transfer the seasoned scallops to the basket, spacing them apart.
4. Put the air fryer basket on the baking pan and slide into Rack Position 2, select Air Fry, set temperature to 390ºF (199ºC), and set time to 4 minutes.
5. Flip the scallops halfway through the cooking time.
6. When cooking is complete, the scallops should reach an internal temperature of just 145ºF (63ºC) on a meat thermometer. Sprinkle the pepper and thyme leaves on top for garnish, if desired. Serve immediately.

200.Air Fried Cod Fillets

Servings:4
Cooking Time: 12 Minutes
Ingredients:
- 4 cod fillets
- ¼ teaspoon fine sea salt
- 1 teaspoon cayenne pepper
- ¼ teaspoon ground black pepper, or more to taste
- ½ cup fresh Italian parsley, coarsely chopped
- ½ cup non-dairy milk
- 4 garlic cloves, minced
- 1 Italian pepper, chopped
- 1 teaspoon dried basil
- ½ teaspoon dried oregano
- Cooking spray

Directions:
1. Lightly spritz the air fryer basket with cooking spray.
2. Season the fillets with salt, cayenne pepper, and black pepper.
3. Pulse the remaining ingredients in a food processor, then transfer the mixture to a shallow bowl. Coat the fillets with the mixture. Place the fillets in the basket.
4. Put the air fryer basket on the baking pan and slide into Rack Position 2, select Air Fry, set temperature to 375ºF (190ºC), and set time to 12 minutes.
5. When cooking is complete, the fish will be flaky. Remove from the oven and serve on a plate.

201.Browned Shrimp Patties

Servings:4
Cooking Time: 12 Minutes
Ingredients:
- ½ pound (227 g) raw shrimp, shelled, deveined, and chopped finely
- 2 cups cooked sushi rice
- ¼ cup chopped red bell pepper
- ¼ cup chopped celery
- ¼ cup chopped green onion
- 2 teaspoons Worcestershire sauce
- ½ teaspoon salt
- ½ teaspoon garlic powder
- ½ teaspoon Old Bay seasoning
- ½ cup plain bread crumbs
- Cooking spray

Directions:
1. Put all the ingredients except the bread crumbs and oil in a large bowl and stir to incorporate.
2. Scoop out the shrimp mixture and shape into 8 equal-sized patties with your hands, no more than ½-inch thick. Roll the patties in the bread crumbs on a plate and spray both sides with cooking spray. Place the patties in the air fryer basket.
3. Put the air fryer basket on the baking pan and slide into Rack Position 2, select Air Fry, set temperature to 390ºF (199ºC), and set time to 12 minutes.
4. Flip the patties halfway through the cooking time.
5. When cooking is complete, the outside should be crispy brown. Divide the patties among four plates and serve warm.

202.Garlic-butter Shrimp With Vegetables

Servings:4
Cooking Time: 15 Minutes
Ingredients:
- 1 pound (454 g) small red potatoes, halved
- 2 ears corn, shucked and cut into rounds, 1 to 1½ inches thick
- 2 tablespoons Old Bay or similar seasoning
- ½ cup unsalted butter, melted
- 1 (12- to 13-ounce / 340- to 369-g) package kielbasa or other smoked sausages

- 3 garlic cloves, minced
- 1 pound (454 g) medium shrimp, peeled and deveined

Directions:
1. Place the potatoes and corn in a large bowl.
2. Stir together the butter and Old Bay seasoning in a small bowl. Drizzle half the butter mixture over the potatoes and corn, tossing to coat. Spread out the vegetables in the baking pan.
3. Slide the baking pan into Rack Position 2, select Roast, set temperature to 350ºF (180ºC), and set time to 15 minutes.
4. Meanwhile, cut the sausages into 2-inch lengths, then cut each piece in half lengthwise. Put the sausages and shrimp in a medium bowl and set aside.
5. Add the garlic to the bowl of remaining butter mixture and stir well.
6. After 10 minutes, remove the pan and pour the vegetables into the large bowl. Drizzle with the garlic butter and toss until well coated. Arrange the vegetables, sausages, and shrimp in the pan.
7. Return to the oven and continue cooking. After 5 minutes, check the shrimp for doneness. The shrimp should be pink and opaque. If they are not quite cooked through, roast for an additional 1 minute.
8. When done, remove from the oven and serve on a plate.

203.Herbed Scallops With Vegetables

Servings:4
Cooking Time: 9 Minutes
Ingredients:
- 1 cup frozen peas
- 1 cup green beans
- 1 cup frozen chopped broccoli
- 2 teaspoons olive oil
- ½ teaspoon dried oregano
- ½ teaspoon dried basil
- 12 ounces (340 g) sea scallops, rinsed and patted dry

Directions:
1. Put the peas, green beans, and broccoli in a large bowl. Drizzle with the olive oil and

toss to coat well. Transfer the vegetables to the air fryer basket.
2. Put the air fryer basket on the baking pan and slide into Rack Position 2, select Air Fry, set temperature to 400ºF (205ºC), and set time to 5 minutes.
3. When cooking is complete, the vegetables should be fork-tender. Transfer the vegetables to a serving bowl. Scatter with the oregano and basil and set aside.
4. Place the scallops in the basket.
5. Put the air fryer basket on the baking pan and slide into Rack Position 2, select Air Fry, set temperature to 400ºF (205ºC), and set time to 4 minutes.
6. When cooking is complete, the scallops should be firm and just opaque in the center. Remove from the oven to the bowl of vegetables and toss well. Serve warm.

204.Air-fried Scallops

Servings:2
Cooking Time: 12 Minutes
Ingredients:
- $1/_3$ cup shallots, chopped
- 1½ tablespoons olive oil
- 1½ tablespoons coconut aminos
- 1 tablespoon Mediterranean seasoning mix
- ½ tablespoon balsamic vinegar
- ½ teaspoon ginger, grated
- 1 clove garlic, chopped
- 1 pound (454 g) scallops, cleanedCooking spray
- Belgian endive, for garnish

Directions:
1. Place all the ingredients except the scallops and Belgian endive in a small skillet over medium heat and stir to combine. Let this mixture simmer for about 2 minutes.
2. Remove the mixture from the skillet to a large bowl and set aside to cool.
3. Add the scallops, coating them all over, then transfer to the refrigerator to marinate for at least 2 hours.
4. When ready, place the scallops in the air fryer basket in a single layer and spray with cooking spray.

5. Put the air fryer basket on the baking pan and slide into Rack Position 2, select Air Fry, set temperature to 345ºF (174ºC), and set time to 10 minutes.
6. Flip the scallops halfway through the cooking time.
7. When cooking is complete, the scallops should be tender and opaque. Remove from the oven and serve garnished with the Belgian endive.

205.Fish Cakes With Mango Relish

Servings: 4
Cooking Time: 10 Minutes
Ingredients:
- 1 lb White Fish Fillets
- 3 Tbsps Ground Coconut
- 1 Ripened Mango
- ½ Tsps Chili Paste
- Tbsps Fresh Parsley
- 1 Green Onion
- 1 Lime
- 1 Tsp Salt
- 1 Egg

Directions:
1. Preparing the Ingredients. To make the relish, peel and dice the mango into cubes. Combine with a half teaspoon of chili paste, a tablespoon of parsley, and the zest and juice of half a lime.
2. In a food processor, pulse the fish until it forms a smooth texture. Place into a bowl and add the salt, egg, chopped green onion, parsley, two tablespoons of the coconut, and the remainder of the chili paste and lime zest and juice. Combine well
3. Portion the mixture into 10 equal balls and flatten them into small patties. Pour the reserved tablespoon of coconut onto a dish and roll the patties over to coat.
4. Preheat the Air fryer oven to 390 degrees
5. Air Frying. Place the fish cakes into the Cuisinart air fryer oven and cook for 8 minutes. They should be crisp and lightly browned when ready
6. Serve hot with mango relish

206.Goat Cheese Shrimp

Servings:2
Cooking Time: 8 Minutes
Ingredients:
- 1 pound (454 g) shrimp, deveined
- 1½ tablespoons olive oil
- 1½ tablespoons balsamic vinegar
- 1 tablespoon coconut aminos
- ½ tablespoon fresh parsley, roughly chopped
- Sea salt flakes, to taste
- 1 teaspoon Dijon mustard
- ½ teaspoon smoked cayenne pepper
- ½ teaspoon garlic powder
- Salt and ground black peppercorns, to taste
- 1 cup shredded goat cheese

Directions:
1. Except for the cheese, stir together all the ingredients in a large bowl until the shrimp are evenly coated.
2. Place the shrimp in the air fryer basket.
3. Put the air fryer basket on the baking pan and slide into Rack Position 2, select Roast, set temperature to 385ºF (196ºC), and set time to 8 minutes.
4. When cooking is complete, the shrimp should be pink and cooked through. Remove from the oven and serve with the shredded goat cheese sprinkled on top.

207.Perfect Crab Cakes

Servings: 6
Cooking Time: 30 Minutes
Ingredients:
- 16 oz lump crab meat
- 1/4 cup celery, diced
- 1/4 cup onion, diced
- 1 cup crushed crackers
- 1 tsp old bay seasoning
- 1 tsp brown mustard
- 2/3 cup mashed avocado

Directions:
1. Fit the Cuisinart oven with the rack in position
2. Add all ingredients into the bowl and mix until just combined.

3. Make small patties from mixture and place in parchment-lined baking pan.
4. Set to bake at 350 F for 35 minutes. After 5 minutes place the baking dish in the preheated oven.
5. Serve and enjoy.
- **Nutrition Info:** Calories 84 Fat 7.7 g Carbohydrates 4.6 g Sugar 0.8 g Protein 11.5 g Cholesterol 43 mg

208.Smoked Paprika Tiger Shrimp

Servings:4
Cooking Time: 10 Minutes
Ingredients:
- 1 lb tiger shrimp
- 2 tbsp olive oil
- ¼ tbsp garlic powder
- 1 tbsp smoked paprika
- 2 tbsp fresh parsley, chopped
- Sea salt to taste

Directions:
1. Preheat Breville on AirFry function to 380 F. Mix garlic powder, smoked paprika, salt, parsley, and olive oil in a large bowl. Add in the shrimp and toss to coat. Place the shrimp in the frying basket press Start. Fry for 6-7 minutes. Serve with salad.

209.Lobster Spicy Lemon Kebab

Servings:x
Cooking Time:x
Ingredients:
- 1 lb. lobster (Shelled and cubed)
- 3 onions chopped
- 5 green chilies-roughly chopped
- 1 ½ tbsp. ginger paste
- 1 ½ tsp garlic paste
- 1 ½ tsp salt
- 3 tsp lemon juice
- 2 tsp garam masala
- 4 tbsp. chopped coriander
- 3 tbsp. cream
- 2 tbsp. coriander powder
- 4 tbsp. fresh mint chopped
- 3 tbsp. chopped capsicum
- 3 eggs
- 2 ½ tbsp. white sesame seeds

Directions:

1. Take all the ingredients mentioned under the first heading and mix them in a bowl. Grind them thoroughly to make a smooth paste.
2. Take the eggs in a different bowl and beat them. Add a pinch of salt and leave them aside.
3. Take a flat plate and in it mix the sesame seeds and breadcrumbs.
4. Dip the lobster cubes in the egg and salt mixture and then in the mixture of
5. breadcrumbs and sesame seeds. Leave these kebabs in the fridge for an hour or so to set.
6. Pre heat the Breville smart oven at 160 degrees Fahrenheit for around 5 minutes. Place the kebabs in the basket and let them cook for another 25 minutes at the same temperature. Turn the kebabs over in between the cooking process to get a uniform cook. Serve the kebabs with mint sauce.

210.Tuna Sandwich

Servings:x
Cooking Time:x
Ingredients:
- 2 slices of white bread
- 1 tbsp. softened butter
- 1 tin tuna
- 1 small capsicum
- For Barbeque Sauce:
- ¼ tbsp. Worcestershire sauce
- ½ tsp. olive oil
- ¼ tsp. mustard powder
- ½ flake garlic crushed
- ¼ cup chopped onion
- ½ tbsp. sugar
- 1 tbsp. tomato ketchup
- ½ cup water.
- ¼ tbsp. red chili sauce
- A pinch of salt and black pepper to taste

Directions:
1. Take the slices of bread and remove the edges. Now cut the slices horizontally. Cook the ingredients for the sauce and wait till it thickens. Now, add the lamb to the sauce and stir till it obtains the flavors. Roast the

capsicum and peel the skin off. Cut the capsicum into slices. Mix the ingredients together and apply it to the bread slices.

2. Pre-heat the Breville smart oven for 5 minutes at 300 Fahrenheit. Open the basket of the Fryer and place the prepared Classic Sandwiches in it such that no two Classic Sandwiches are touching each other. Now keep the fryer at 250 degrees for around 15 minutes. Turn the Classic Sandwiches in between the cooking process to cook both slices. Serve the Classic Sandwiches with tomato ketchup or mint sauce.

211. Marinated Salmon

Servings: 2
Cooking Time: 10 Minutes
Ingredients:
- 2 salmon fillets, skinless and boneless
- For marinade:
- 2 tbsp scallions, minced
- 1 tbsp ginger, grated
- 2 garlic cloves, minced
- 2 tbsp mirin
- 2 tbsp soy sauce
- 1 tbsp olive oil

Directions:
1. Fit the Cuisinart oven with the rack in position 2.
2. Add all marinade ingredients into the zip-lock bag and mix well.
3. Add salmon in the bag. The sealed bag shakes well and places it in the fridge for 30 minutes.
4. Arrange marinated salmon fillets in an air fryer basket then place an air fryer basket in the baking pan.
5. Place a baking pan on the oven rack. Set to air fry at 360 F for 10 minutes.
6. Serve and enjoy.
- **Nutrition Info:** Calories 345 Fat 18.2 g Carbohydrates 11.6 g Sugar 4.5 g Protein 36.1 g Cholesterol 78 mg

212. Dijon Salmon Fillets

Servings: 4
Cooking Time: 15 Minutes
Ingredients:
- 1 lb salmon fillets
- 2 tbsp Dijon mustard
- 1/4 cup brown sugar
- Pepper
- Salt

Directions:
1. Fit the Cuisinart oven with the rack in position 2.
2. Season salmon fillets with pepper and salt.
3. In a small bowl, mix Dijon mustard and brown sugar.
4. Brush salmon fillets with Dijon mustard mixture.
5. Place salmon fillets in the air fryer basket then place an air fryer basket in the baking pan.
6. Place a baking pan on the oven rack. Set to air fry at 350 F for 15 minutes.
7. Serve and enjoy.
- **Nutrition Info:** Calories 190 Fat 7.3 g Carbohydrates 9.3 g Sugar 8.9 g Protein 22.4 g Cholesterol 50 mg

213. Tasty Parmesan Shrimp

Servings: 4
Cooking Time: 10 Minutes
Ingredients:
- 1 lb shrimp, peeled and deveined
- 1/4 cup parmesan cheese, grated
- 4 garlic cloves, minced
- 1 tbsp olive oil
- 1/4 tsp oregano
- 1/2 tsp pepper
- 1/2 tsp onion powder
- 1/2 tsp basil

Directions:
1. Fit the Cuisinart oven with the rack in position 2.
2. Add all ingredients into the large bowl and toss well.
3. Add shrimp to the air fryer basket then place an air fryer basket in the baking pan.
4. Place a baking pan on the oven rack. Set to air fry at 350 F for 10 minutes.
5. Serve and enjoy.
- **Nutrition Info:** Calories 189 Fat 6.7 g Carbohydrates 3.4 g Sugar 0.1 g Protein 27.9 g Cholesterol 243 mg

214.Sesame Seeds Coated Fish

Servings:5
Cooking Time: 8 Minutes
Ingredients:

- 3 tablespoons plain flour
- 2 eggs
- ½ cup sesame seeds, toasted
- ½ cup breadcrumbs
- 1/8 teaspoon dried rosemary, crushed
- Pinch of salt
- Pinch of black pepper
- 3 tablespoons olive oil
- 5 frozen fish fillets (white fish of your choice)

Directions:

1. Preparing the Ingredients. In a shallow dish, place flour. In a second shallow dish, beat the eggs. In a third shallow dish, add remaining ingredients except fish fillets and mix till a crumbly mixture forms.
2. Coat the fillets with flour and shake off the excess flour.
3. Next, dip the fillets in the egg.
4. Then coat the fillets with sesame seeds mixture generously.
5. Preheat the Cuisinart air fryer oven to 390 degrees F.
6. Air Frying. Line an Air fryer rack/basket with a piece of foil. Arrange the fillets into prepared basket.
7. Cook for about 14 minutes, flipping once after 10 minutes.

215.Rosemary Garlic Shrimp

Servings: 4
Cooking Time: 10 Minutes
Ingredients:

- 1 lb shrimp, peeled and deveined
- 2 garlic cloves, minced
- 1/2 tbsp fresh rosemary, chopped
- 1 tbsp olive oil
- Pepper
- Salt

Directions:

1. Fit the Cuisinart oven with the rack in position

2. Add shrimp and remaining ingredients in a large bowl and toss well.
3. Pour shrimp mixture into the baking dish.
4. Set to bake at 400 F for 15 minutes. After 5 minutes place the baking dish in the preheated oven.
5. Serve and enjoy.
- **Nutrition Info:** Calories 168 Fat 5.5 g Carbohydrates 2.5 g Sugar 0 g Protein 26 g Cholesterol 239 mg

216.Old Bay Tilapia Fillets

Servings: 4
Cooking Time: 15 Minutes
Ingredients:

- 1 pound tilapia fillets
- 1 tbsp old bay seasoning
- 2 tbsp canola oil
- 2 tbsp lemon pepper
- Salt to taste
- 2-3 butter buds

Directions:

1. Preheat your Cuisinart oven to 400 F on Bake function. Drizzle tilapia fillets with canola oil. In a bowl, mix salt, lemon pepper, butter buds, and seasoning; spread on the fish. Place the fillet on the basket and fit in the baking tray. Cook for 10 minutes, flipping once until tender and crispy.

217.Baked Spinach Tilapia

Servings: 4
Cooking Time: 10 Minutes
Ingredients:

- 1 lb tilapia fillets
- 1 cup Monterey jack cheese, shredded
- 3 tbsp butter, sliced
- 8 oz spinach

Directions:

1. Fit the Cuisinart oven with the rack in position
2. Add spinach into the baking dish and top with butter slices.
3. Place fish fillets on top of spinach.
4. Sprinkle shredded cheese over fish fillets.
5. Set to bake at 450 F for 15 minutes. After 5 minutes place the baking dish in the preheated oven.

6. Serve and enjoy.
- **Nutrition Info:** Calories 288 Fat 18.4 g Carbohydrates 2.3 g Sugar 0.4 g Protein 29.7 g Cholesterol 103 mg

218.Air Fryer Salmon

Servings: 2
Cooking Time: 10 Minutes
Ingredients:
- ½ tsp. salt
- ½ tsp. garlic powder
- ½ tsp. smoked paprika
- Salmon

Directions:
1. Preparing the Ingredients. Mix spices and sprinkle onto salmon.
2. Place seasoned salmon into the Cuisinart air fryer oven.
3. Air Frying. Set temperature to 400°F, and set time to 10 minutes.
- **Nutrition Info:** CALORIES: 185; FAT: 11G; PROTEIN:21G; SUGAR:0G

219.Garlicky Cod Fillets

Servings:4
Cooking Time: 12 Minutes
Ingredients:
- 1 teaspoon olive oil
- 4 cod fillets
- ¼ teaspoon fine sea salt
- ¼ teaspoon ground black pepper, or more to taste
- 1 teaspoon cayenne pepper
- ½ cup fresh Italian parsley, coarsely chopped
- ½ cup nondairy milk
- 1 Italian pepper, chopped
- 4 garlic cloves, minced
- 1 teaspoon dried basil
- ½ teaspoon dried oregano

Directions:
1. Lightly coat the sides and bottom of the baking pan with the olive oil. Set aside.
2. In a large bowl, sprinkle the fillets with salt, black pepper, and cayenne pepper.
3. In a food processor, pulse the remaining ingredients until smoothly puréed.

4. Add the purée to the bowl of fillets and toss to coat, then transfer to the prepared baking pan.
5. Slide the baking pan into Rack Position 1, select Convection Bake, set temperature to 380ºF (193ºC), and set time to 12 minutes.
6. When cooking is complete, the fish should flake when pressed lightly with a fork. Remove from the oven and serve warm.

220.Cajun Red Snapper

Servings: 2
Cooking Time: 12 Minutes
Ingredients:
- 8 oz red snapper fillets
- 2 tbsp parmesan cheese, grated
- 1/4 cup breadcrumbs
- 1/2 tsp Cajun seasoning
- 1/4 tsp Worcestershire sauce
- 1 garlic clove, minced
- 1/4 cup butter

Directions:
1. Fit the Cuisinart oven with the rack in position
2. Melt butter in a pan over low heat. Add Cajun seasoning, garlic, and Worcestershire sauce into the melted butter and stir well.
3. Brush fish fillets with melted butter and place into the baking dish.
4. Mix together parmesan cheese and breadcrumbs and sprinkle over fish fillets.
5. Set to bake at 400 F for 17 minutes. After 5 minutes place the baking dish in the preheated oven.
6. Serve and enjoy.
- **Nutrition Info:** Calories 424 Fat 27 g Carbohydrates 10.6 g Sugar 1 g Protein 33.9 g Cholesterol 119 mg

221.Crab Cakes With Bell Peppers

Servings:4
Cooking Time: 10 Minutes
Ingredients:
- 8 ounces (227 g) jumbo lump crab meat
- 1 egg, beaten
- Juice of ½ lemon
- $^1/_3$ cup bread crumbs
- ¼ cup diced green bell pepper

- ¼ cup diced red bell pepper
- ¼ cup mayonnaise
- 1 tablespoon Old Bay seasoning
- 1 teaspoon flour
- Cooking spray

Directions:

1. Make the crab cakes: Place all the ingredients except the flour and oil in a large bowl and stir until well incorporated.
2. Divide the crab mixture into four equal portions and shape each portion into a patty with your hands. Top each patty with a sprinkle of ¼ teaspoon of flour.
3. Arrange the crab cakes in the air fryer basket and spritz them with cooking spray.
4. Put the air fryer basket on the baking pan and slide into Rack Position 2, select Air Fry, set temperature to 375ºF (190ºC), and set time to 10 minutes.
5. Flip the crab cakes halfway through.
6. When cooking is complete, the cakes should be cooked through. Remove from the oven and divide the crab cakes among four plates and serve.

222.Baked Garlic Tilapia

Servings: 4
Cooking Time: 15 Minutes
Ingredients:

- 1 lb tilapia fillets
- 2 tbsp garlic, minced
- 2 tbsp olive oil
- 2 tbsp dried parsley
- Pepper
- Salt

Directions:

1. Fit the Cuisinart oven with the rack in position
2. Place fish fillets in a baking dish. Drizzle with oil and season with pepper and salt.
3. Sprinkle garlic and parsley over fish fillets.
4. Set to bake at 400 F for 20 minutes. After 5 minutes place the baking dish in the preheated oven.
5. Serve and enjoy.
- **Nutrition Info:** Calories 160 Fat 8.1 g Carbohydrates 1.5 g Sugar 0.1 g Protein 21.4 g Cholesterol 55 mg

223.Lemon Pepper Tilapia Fillets

Servings:4
Cooking Time: 15 Minutes
Ingredients:

- 1 lb tilapia fillets
- 1 tbsp Italian seasoning
- 2 tbsp canola oil
- 2 tbsp lemon pepper
- Salt to taste
- 2-3 butter buds

Directions:

1. Preheat your Breville oven to 400 F on Bake function. Drizzle tilapia fillets with canola oil. In a bowl, mix salt, lemon pepper, butter buds, and Italian seasoning; spread on the fish. Place the fillet on a baking tray and press Start. Cook for 10 minutes until tender and crispy. Serve warm.

224.Fried Cod Nuggets

Servings: 4
Cooking Time: 25 Minutes
Ingredients:

- 1 ¼ lb cod fillets, cut into 4 to 6 chunks each
- ½ cup flour
- 1 egg
- 1 cup cornflakes
- 1 tbsp olive oil
- Salt and black pepper to taste

Directions:

1. Place the olive oil and cornflakes in a food processor and process until crumbed. Season the fish chunks with salt and pepper. In a bowl, beat the egg along with 1 tbsp of water. Dredge the chunks in flour first, then dip in the egg, and finally coat with cornflakes. Arrange the fish pieces on a lined sheet and cook in your Cuisinart on Air Fry at 350 F for 15 minutes until crispy.

225.Tomato Garlic Shrimp

Servings: 4
Cooking Time: 25 Minutes
Ingredients:

- 1 lb shrimp, peeled
- 1 tbsp garlic, sliced
- 2 cups cherry tomatoes

- 1 tbsp olive oil
- Pepper
- Salt

Directions:
1. Fit the Cuisinart oven with the rack in position
2. Add shrimp, oil, garlic, tomatoes, pepper, and salt into the large bowl and toss well.
3. Transfer shrimp mixture into the baking dish.
4. Set to bake at 400 F for 30 minutes. After 5 minutes place the baking dish in the preheated oven.
5. Serve and enjoy.
- **Nutrition Info:** Calories 184 Fat 5.6 g Carbohydrates 5.9 g Sugar 2.4 g Protein 26.8 gCholesterol 239 mg

226.Spinach Scallops

Servings: 2
Cooking Time: 10 Minutes
Ingredients:
- 8 sea scallops
- 1 tbsp fresh basil, chopped
- 1 tbsp tomato paste
- 3/4 cup heavy cream
- 12 oz frozen spinach, thawed and drained
- 1 tsp garlic, minced
- 1/2 tsp pepper
- 1/2 tsp salt

Directions:
1. Fit the Cuisinart oven with the rack in position
2. Layer spinach in the baking dish.
3. Spray scallops with cooking spray and season with pepper and salt.
4. Place scallops on top of spinach.
5. In a small bowl, mix garlic, basil, tomato paste, whipping cream, pepper, and salt and pour over scallops and spinach.
6. Set to bake at 350 F for 15 minutes. After 5 minutes place the baking dish in the preheated oven.
7. Serve and enjoy.
- **Nutrition Info:** Calories 310 Fat 18.3 g Carbohydrates 12.6 g Sugar 1.7 g Protein 26.5 g Cholesterol 101 mg

227.Prawn Fried Baked Pastry

Servings:x
Cooking Time:x
Ingredients:
- 2 tbsp. unsalted butter
- 1 ½ cup all-purpose flour
- A pinch of salt to taste
- Add as much water as required to make the dough stiff and firm
- 1 lb. prawn
- ¼ cup boiled peas
- 1 tsp. powdered ginger
- 1 or 2 green chilies that are finely chopped or mashed
- ½ tsp. cumin
- 1 tsp. coarsely crushed coriander
- 1 dry red chili broken into pieces
- A small amount of salt (to taste)
- ½ tsp. dried mango powder
- ½ tsp. red chili power.
- 1-2 tbsp. coriander.

Directions:
1. You will first need to make the outer covering. In a large bowl, add the flour, butter and enough water to knead it into dough that is stiff. Transfer this to a container and leave it to rest for five minutes. Place a pan on medium flame and add the oil. Roast the mustard seeds and once roasted, add the coriander seeds and the chopped dry red chilies. Add all the dry ingredients for the filling and mix the ingredients well.
2. Add a little water and continue to stir the ingredients. Make small balls out of the dough and roll them out. Cut the rolled-out dough into halves and apply a little water on the edges to help you fold the halves into a cone. Add the filling to the cone and close up the samosa. Pre-heat the Breville smart oven for around 5 to 6 minutes at 300 Fahrenheit. Place all the samosas in the fry basket and close the basket properly.
3. Keep the Breville smart oven at 200 degrees for another 20 to 25 minutes. Around the halfway point, open the basket and turn the samosas over for uniform cooking. After

this, fry at 250 degrees for around 10 minutes in order to give them the desired golden-brown color. Serve hot. Recommended sides are tamarind or mint sauce.

228.Coconut Shrimp

Servings: 4
Cooking Time: 5 Minutes
Ingredients:

- 1 (8-ounce) can crushed pineapple
- ½ cup sour cream
- ¼ cup pineapple preserves
- 2 egg whites
- ⅔ cup cornstarch
- ⅔ cup sweetened coconut
- 1 cup panko bread crumbs
- 1 pound uncooked large shrimp, thawed if frozen, deveined and shelled
- Olive oil for misting

Directions:

1. Preparing the Ingredients. Drain the crushed pineapple well, reserving the juice. In a small bowl, combine the pineapple, sour cream, and preserves, and mix well. Set aside. In a shallow bowl, beat the egg whites with 2 tablespoons of the reserved pineapple liquid. Place the cornstarch on a plate. Combine the coconut and bread crumbs on another plate. Dip the shrimp into the cornstarch, shake it off, then dip into the egg white mixture and finally into the coconut mixture. Place the shrimp in the air fryer rack/basket and mist with oil.
2. Air Frying. Air-fry for 5 to 7 minutes or until the shrimp are crisp and golden brown.
- **Nutrition Info:** CALORIES: 524; FAT: 14G; PROTEIN:33G; FIBER:4G

229.Parmesan Fish Fillets

Servings:4
Cooking Time: 17 Minutes
Ingredients:

- $^1/_3$ cup grated Parmesan cheese
- ½ teaspoon fennel seed
- ½ teaspoon tarragon
- $^1/_3$ teaspoon mixed peppercorns
- 2 eggs, beaten

- 4 (4-ounce / 113-g) fish fillets, halved
- 2 tablespoons dry white wine
- 1 teaspoon seasoned salt

Directions:

1. Place the grated Parmesan cheese, fennel seed, tarragon, and mixed peppercorns in a food processor and pulse for about 20 seconds until well combined. Transfer the cheese mixture to a shallow dish.
2. Place the beaten eggs in another shallow dish.
3. Drizzle the dry white wine over the top of fish fillets. Dredge each fillet in the beaten eggs on both sides, shaking off any excess, then roll them in the cheese mixture until fully coated. Season with the salt.
4. Arrange the fillets in the air fryer basket.
5. Put the air fryer basket on the baking pan and slide into Rack Position 2, select Air Fry, set temperature to 345ºF (174ºC), and set time to 17 minutes.
6. Flip the fillets once halfway through the cooking time.
7. When cooking is complete, the fish should be cooked through no longer translucent. Remove from the oven and cool for 5 minutes before serving.

230.Carp Best Homemade Croquette

Servings:x
Cooking Time:x
Ingredients:

- 1 lb. Carp filets
- 3 onions chopped
- 5 green chilies-roughly chopped
- 1 ½ tbsp. ginger paste
- 1 ½ tsp garlic paste
- 1 ½ tsp salt
- 3 tsp lemon juice
- 2 tsp garam masala
- 4 tbsp. chopped coriander
- 3 tbsp. cream
- 2 tbsp. coriander powder
- 4 tbsp. fresh mint chopped
- 3 tbsp. chopped capsicum
- 3 eggs
- 2 ½ tbsp. white sesame seeds

Directions:

1. Take all the ingredients mentioned under the first heading and mix them in a bowl. Grind them thoroughly to make a smooth paste. Take the eggs in a different bowl and beat them. Add a pinch of salt and leave them aside. Mold the fish mixture into small balls and flatten them into round and flat Best Homemade Croquettes. Dip these Best Homemade Croquettes in the egg and salt mixture and then in the mixture of breadcrumbs and sesame seeds.

2. Leave these Best Homemade Croquettes in the fridge for an hour or so to set. Pre heat the Breville smart oven at 160 degrees Fahrenheit for around 5 minutes. Place the Best Homemade Croquettes in the basket and let them cook for another 25 minutes at the same temperature. Turn the Best Homemade Croquettes over in between the cooking process to get a uniform cook. Serve the Best Homemade Croquettes with mint sauce.

231. Lemon Pepper White Fish Fillets

Servings: 2
Cooking Time: 12 Minutes
Ingredients:
- 12 oz white fish fillets
- 1/2 tsp lemon pepper seasoning
- Pepper
- Salt

Directions:
1. Fit the Cuisinart oven with the rack in position 2.
2. Spray fish fillets with cooking spray and season with lemon pepper seasoning, pepper, and salt.
3. Place fish fillets in the air fryer basket then place an air fryer basket in the baking pan.
4. Place a baking pan on the oven rack. Set to air fry at 360 F for 12 minutes.
5. Serve and enjoy.
- **Nutrition Info:** Calories 294 Fat 12.8 g Carbohydrates 0.4 g Sugar 0 g Protein 41.7 g Cholesterol 131 mg

232. Tilapia Meunière With Vegetables

Servings: 4

Cooking Time: 20 Minutes
Ingredients:
- 10 ounces (283 g) Yukon Gold potatoes, sliced ¼-inch thick
- 5 tablespoons unsalted butter, melted, divided
- 1 teaspoon kosher salt, divided
- 4 (8-ounce / 227-g) tilapia fillets
- ½ pound (227 g) green beans, trimmed
- Juice of 1 lemon
- 2 tablespoons chopped fresh parsley, for garnish

Directions:
1. In a large bowl, drizzle the potatoes with 2 tablespoons of melted butter and ¼ teaspoon of kosher salt. Transfer the potatoes to the baking pan.
2. Slide the baking pan into Rack Position 2, select Roast, set temperature to 375ºF (190ºC), and set time to 20 minutes.
3. Meanwhile, season both sides of the fillets with ½ teaspoon of kosher salt. Put the green beans in the medium bowl and sprinkle with the remaining ¼ teaspoon of kosher salt and 1 tablespoon of butter, tossing to coat.
4. After 10 minutes, remove from the oven and push the potatoes to one side. Put the fillets in the middle of the pan and add the green beans on the other side. Drizzle the remaining 2 tablespoons of butter over the fillets. Return the pan to the oven and continue cooking, or until the fish flakes easily with a fork and the green beans are crisp-tender.
5. When cooked, remove from the oven. Drizzle the lemon juice over the fillets and sprinkle the parsley on top for garnish. Serve hot.

233. Blackened Mahi Mahi

Servings: 4
Cooking Time: 12 Minutes
Ingredients:
- 4 mahi-mahi fillets
- 1 tsp cumin
- 1 tsp paprika
- 1/2 tsp cayenne pepper

- 1 tsp oregano
- 1 tsp garlic powder
- 1 tsp onion powder
- 1/2 tsp pepper
- 3 tbsp olive oil
- 1/2 tsp salt

Directions:

1. Fit the Cuisinart oven with the rack in position
2. Brush fish fillets with oil and place them into the baking dish.
3. Mix together the remaining ingredients and sprinkle over fish fillets.
4. Set to bake at 450 F for 17 minutes. After 5 minutes place the baking dish in the preheated oven.
5. Serve and enjoy.
- **Nutrition Info:** Calories 189 Fat 11.7 g Carbohydrates 2.1 g Sugar 0.5 g Protein 19.4 g Cholesterol 86 mg

234.Dill Salmon Patties

Servings: 2
Cooking Time: 10 Minutes

Ingredients:

- 14 oz can salmon, drained and discard bones
- 1 tsp dill, chopped
- 1 egg, lightly beaten
- 1/4 tsp garlic powder
- 1/2 cup breadcrumbs
- 1/4 cup onion, diced
- Pepper
- Salt

Directions:

1. Fit the Cuisinart oven with the rack in position 2.
2. Add all ingredients into the large bowl and mix well.
3. Make equal shapes of patties from mixture and place in the air fryer basket then place the air fryer basket in the baking pan.
4. Place a baking pan on the oven rack. Set to air fry at 370 F for 10 minutes.
5. Serve and enjoy.
- **Nutrition Info:** Calories 422 Fat 15.7 g Carbohydrates 21.5 g Sugar 2.5 g Protein 46 g Cholesterol 191 mg

MEATLESS RECIPES

235.Easy Cheesy Vegetable Quesadilla

Servings:1
Cooking Time: 10 Minutes
Ingredients:

- 1 teaspoon olive oil
- 2 flour tortillas
- ¼ zucchini, sliced
- ¼ yellow bell pepper, sliced
- ¼ cup shredded gouda cheese
- 1 tablespoon chopped cilantro
- ½ green onion, sliced

Directions:

1. Coat the air fryer basket with 1 teaspoon of olive oil.
2. Arrange a flour tortilla in the basket and scatter the top with zucchini, bell pepper, gouda cheese, cilantro, and green onion. Place the other flour tortilla on top.
3. Put the air fryer basket on the baking pan and slide into Rack Position 2, select Air Fry, set temperature to 390ºF (199ºC), and set time to 10 minutes.
4. When cooking is complete, the tortillas should be lightly browned and the vegetables should be tender. Remove from the oven and cool for 5 minutes before slicing into wedges.

236.Zucchini Parmesan Crisps

Servings: 4
Cooking Time: 25 Minutes
Ingredients:

- 4 small zucchini, cut lengthwise
- ½ cup Parmesan cheese, grated
- ½ cup breadcrumbs
- ¼ cup melted butter
- ¼ cup chopped parsley
- 4 garlic cloves, minced
- Salt and black pepper to taste

Directions:

1. Preheat Cuisinart on Air Fry function to 350 F. In a bowl, mix breadcrumbs, Parmesan cheese, garlic, parsley, salt, and pepper. Stir in butter. Place the zucchinis cut-side up in a baking tray.

2. Spread the cheese mixture onto the zucchini evenly. Cook for 13 minutes. Increase the temperature to 370 F and cook for 3 more minutes for extra crunchiness. Serve hot.

237.Mushroom Fried Baked Pastry

Servings:x
Cooking Time:x
Ingredients:

- 2 capsicum sliced
- 2 carrot sliced
- 2 cabbage sliced
- 2 tbsp. soya sauce
- 2 tsp. vinegar
- 1 cup all-purpose flour
- 2 tbsp. unsalted butter
- A pinch of salt to taste
- Take the amount of water sufficient enough to make a stiff dough
- 3 cups whole mushrooms
- 2 onion sliced
- 2 tbsp. green chilies finely chopped
- 2 tbsp. ginger-garlic paste
- Some salt and pepper to taste

Directions:

1. Mix the dough for the outer covering and make it stiff and smooth. Leave it to rest in a container while making the filling.
2. Cook the ingredients in a pan and stir them well to make a thick paste. Roll the paste out.
3. Roll the dough into balls and flatten them. Cut them in halves and add the filling. Use water to help you fold the edges to create the shape of a cone.
4. Pre-heat the Breville smart oven for around 5 to 6 minutes at 300 Fahrenheit. Place all the samosas in the fry basket and close the basket properly. Keep the Breville smart oven at 200 degrees for another 20 to 25 minutes. Around the halfway point, open the basket and turn the samosas over for uniform cooking. After this, fry at 250 degrees for around 10 minutes in order to give them the desired golden-brown color. Serve hot. Recommended sides are tamarind or mint sauce.

238.Vegetable Skewer

Servings:x
Cooking Time:x
Ingredients:
- 3 tbsp. cream
- 3 eggs
- 2 cups mixed vegetables
- 3 onions chopped
- 5 green chilies
- 1 ½ tbsp. ginger paste
- 1 ½ tsp. garlic paste
- 1 ½ tsp. salt
- 2 ½ tbsp. white sesame seeds

Directions:
1. Grind the ingredients except for the egg and form a smooth paste. Coat the vegetables in the paste. Now, beat the eggs and add a little salt to it.
2. Dip the coated vegetables in the egg mixture and then transfer to the sesame seeds and coat the vegetables well. Place the vegetables on a stick.
3. Pre heat the Breville smart oven at 160 degrees Fahrenheit for around 5 minutes. Place the sticks in the basket and let them cook for another 25 minutes at the same temperature. Turn the sticks over in between the cooking process to get a uniform cook.

239.Potato Wedges

Servings:x
Cooking Time:x
Ingredients:
- 1 tsp. mixed herbs
- ½ tsp. red chili flakes
- A pinch of salt to taste
- 1 tbsp. lemon juice
- 2 medium sized potatoes (Cut into wedges)
- ingredients for the marinade:
- 1 tbsp. olive oil

Directions:
1. Boil the potatoes and blanch them. Mix the ingredients for the marinade and add the potato Oregano Fingers to it making sure that they are coated well.

2. Pre heat the Breville smart oven for around 5 minutes at 300 Fahrenheit. Take out the basket of the fryer and place the potato Oregano Fingers in them. Close the basket.
3. Now keep the fryer at 200 Fahrenheit for 20 or 25 minutes. In between the process, toss the fries twice or thrice so that they get cooked properly.

240.Mint French Cuisine Galette

Servings:x
Cooking Time:x
Ingredients:
- 1-2 tbsp. fresh coriander leaves
- 2 or 3 green chilies finely chopped
- 1 ½ tbsp. lemon juice
- Salt and pepper to taste
- 2 cups mint leaves (Sliced fine)
- 2 medium potatoes boiled and mashed
- 1 ½ cup coarsely crushed peanuts
- 3 tsp. ginger finely chopped

Directions:
1. Mix the sliced mint leaves with the rest of the ingredients in a clean bowl.
2. Mold this mixture into round and flat French Cuisine Galettes.
3. Wet the French Cuisine Galettes slightly with water. Coat each French Cuisine Galette with the crushed peanuts.
4. Pre heat the Breville smart oven at 160 degrees Fahrenheit for 5 minutes. Place the French Cuisine Galettes in the fry basket and let them cook for another 25 minutes at the same temperature. Keep rolling them over to get a uniform cook. Serve either with mint sauce or ketchup.

241.Spaghetti Squash Lasagna

Servings: 4
Cooking Time: 15 Minutes
Ingredients:
- 3 lb. spaghetti squash, halved lengthwise & seeded
- 4 tbsp. water, divided
- 1 tbsp. extra-virgin olive oil
- 1 bunch broccolini, chopped
- 4 cloves garlic, chopped fine
- ¼ tsp crushed red pepper flakes

- 1 cup mozzarella cheese, grated &divided
- ¼ cup parmesan cheese, grated & divided
- ¾ tsp Italian seasoning
- ½ tsp salt
- ¼ tsp ground pepper

Directions:

1. Place squash, cut side down, in a microwave safe dish. Add 2 tablespoons water and microwave on high until tender, about 10 minutes.
2. Heat oil in a large skillet over medium heat. Add broccoli, garlic, and red pepper. Cook, stirring frequently, 2 minutes.
3. Add remaining water and cook until broccolini is tender, about 3-5 minutes. Transfer to a large bowl.
4. With a fork, scrape the squash from the shells into the bowl with the broccolini. Place the shells in an 8x11-inch baking pan.
5. Add ¾ cup mozzarella, 2 tablespoons parmesan, and seasonings to the squash mixture and stir to combine. Spoon evenly into the shells and top with remaining cheese.
6. Place rack in position 1 and set oven to bake on 450°F for 15 minutes. After 5 minutes, place the squash in the oven and cook 10 minutes.
7. Set the oven to broil on high and move the pan to position 2. Broil until cheese starts to brown, about 2 minutes. Serve immediately.

- **Nutrition Info:** Calories 328, Total Fat 6g, Saturated Fat 2g, Total Carbs 48g, Net Carbs 39g, Protein 18g, Sugar 3g, Fiber 9g, Sodium 674mg, Potassium 1714mg, Phosphorus 452mg

242.Lemony Brussels Sprouts And Tomatoes

Servings:4
Cooking Time: 20 Minutes
Ingredients:

- 1 pound (454 g) Brussels sprouts, trimmed and halved
- 1 tablespoon extra-virgin olive oil
- Sea Salt and freshly ground black pepper, to taste
- ½ cup sun-dried tomatoes, chopped

- 2 tablespoons freshly squeezed lemon juice
- 1 teaspoon lemon zest

Directions:

1. Line the air fryer basket with aluminum foil.
2. Toss the Brussels sprouts with the olive oil in a large bowl. Sprinkle with salt and black pepper.
3. Spread the Brussels sprouts in a single layer in the basket.
4. Put the air fryer basket on the baking pan and slide into Rack Position 2, select Roast, set temperature to 400ºF (205ºC), and set time to 20 minutes.
5. When done, the Brussels sprouts should be caramelized. Remove from the oven to a serving bowl, along with the tomatoes, lemon juice, and lemon zest. Toss to combine. Serve immediately.

243.Broccoli Momo's Recipe

Servings:x
Cooking Time:x
Ingredients:

- 2 tbsp. oil
- 2 tsp. ginger-garlic paste
- 2 tsp. soya sauce
- 2 tsp. vinegar
- 1 ½ cup all-purpose flour
- ½ tsp. salt
- 5 tbsp. water
- 2 cups grated broccoli

Directions:

1. Squeeze the dough and cover it with plastic wrap and set aside. Next, cook the ingredients for the filling and try to ensure that the broccoli is covered well with the sauce.
2. Roll the dough and cut it into a square. Place the filling in the center. Now, wrap the dough to cover the filling and pinch the edges together.
3. Pre heat the Breville smart oven at 200° F for 5 minutes. Place the gnocchi's in the fry basket and close it. Let them cook at the same temperature for another 20 minutes. Recommended sides are chili sauce or ketchup.

244.Garlic Stuffed Mushrooms

Servings:2
Cooking Time: 12 Minutes
Ingredients:

- 18 medium-sized white mushrooms
- 1 small onion, peeled and chopped
- 4 garlic cloves, peeled and minced
- 2 tablespoons olive oil
- 2 teaspoons cumin powder
- A pinch ground allspice
- Fine sea salt and freshly ground black pepper, to taste

Directions:

1. On a clean work surface, remove the mushroom stems. Using a spoon, scoop out the mushroom gills and discard.
2. Thoroughly combine the onion, garlic, olive oil, cumin powder, allspice, salt, and pepper in a mixing bowl. Stuff the mushrooms evenly with the mixture.
3. Place the stuffed mushrooms in the air fryer basket.
4. Put the air fryer basket on the baking pan and slide into Rack Position 2, select Roast, set temperature to 345ºF (174ºC) and set time to 12 minutes.
5. When cooking is complete, the mushroom should be browned.
6. Cool for 5 minutes before serving.

245.Cheesy Asparagus And Potato Platter

Servings:5
Cooking Time: 26 Minutes
Ingredients:

- 4 medium potatoes, cut into wedges
- Cooking spray
- 1 bunch asparagus, trimmed
- 2 tablespoons olive oil
- Salt and pepper, to taste
- Cheese Sauce:
- ¼ cup crumbled cottage cheese
- ¼ cup buttermilk
- 1 tablespoon whole-grain mustard
- Salt and black pepper, to taste

Directions:

1. Spritz the air fryer basket with cooking spray.
2. Put the potatoes in the air fryer basket.
3. Put the air fryer basket on the baking pan and slide into Rack Position 2, select Roast, set temperature to 400ºF (205ºC) and set time to 20 minutes.
4. Stir the potatoes halfway through.
5. When cooking is complete, the potatoes should be golden brown.
6. Remove the potatoes from the oven to a platter. Cover the potatoes with foil to keep warm. Set aside.
7. Place the asparagus in the air fryer basket and drizzle with the olive oil. Sprinkle with salt and pepper.
8. Put the air fryer basket on the baking pan and slide into Rack Position 2, select Roast, set temperature to 400ºF (205ºC) and set time to 6 minutes. Stir the asparagus halfway through.
9. When cooking is complete, the asparagus should be crispy.
10. Meanwhile, make the cheese sauce by stirring together the cottage cheese, buttermilk, and mustard in a small bowl. Season as needed with salt and pepper.
11. Transfer the asparagus to the platter of potatoes and drizzle with the cheese sauce. Serve immediately.

246.Crispy Veggies With Halloumi

Servings:2
Cooking Time: 14 Minutes
Ingredients:

- 2 zucchinis, cut into even chunks
- 1 large eggplant, peeled, cut into chunks
- 1 large carrot, cut into chunks
- 6 ounces (170 g) halloumi cheese, cubed
- 2 teaspoons olive oil
- Salt and black pepper, to taste
- 1 teaspoon dried mixed herbs

Directions:

1. Combine the zucchinis, eggplant, carrot, cheese, olive oil, salt, and pepper in a large bowl and toss to coat well.
2. Spread the mixture evenly in the air fryer basket.
3. Put the air fryer basket on the baking pan and slide into Rack Position 2, select Air Fry,

set temperature to 340ºF (171ºC), and set time to 14 minutes.

4. Stir the mixture once during cooking.

5. When cooking is complete, they should be crispy and golden. Remove from the oven and serve topped with mixed herbs.

247.Cottage Cheese Fingers

Servings:x
Cooking Time:x
Ingredients:
- 2 tsp. salt
- 1 tsp. pepper powder
- 1 tsp. red chili powder
- 6 tbsp. corn flour
- 4 eggs
- 2 cups cottage cheese Oregano Fingers
- 2 cup dry breadcrumbs
- 2 tsp. oregano
- 1 ½ tbsp. ginger-garlic paste
- 4 tbsp. lemon juice

Directions:
1. Mix all the ingredients for the marinade and put the chicken Oregano Fingers inside and let it rest overnight.
2. Mix the breadcrumbs, oregano and red chili flakes well and place the marinated Oregano Fingers on this mixture. Cover it with plastic wrap and leave it till right before you serve to cook.
3. Pre heat the Breville smart oven at 160 degrees Fahrenheit for 5 minutes. Place the Oregano Fingers in the fry basket and close it. Let them cook at the same temperature for another 15 minutes or so. Toss the Oregano Fingers well so that they are cooked uniformly.

248.Roasted Vegetables With Rice

Servings:4
Cooking Time: 12 Minutes
Ingredients:
- 2 teaspoons melted butter
- 1 cup chopped mushrooms
- 1 cup cooked rice
- 1 cup peas
- 1 carrot, chopped
- 1 red onion, chopped

- 1 garlic clove, minced
- Salt and black pepper, to taste
- 2 hard-boiled eggs, grated
- 1 tablespoon soy sauce

Directions:
1. Coat the baking pan with melted butter.
2. Stir together the mushrooms, cooked rice, peas, carrot, onion, garlic, salt, and pepper in a large bowl until well mixed. Pour the mixture into the prepared baking pan.
3. Slide the baking pan into Rack Position 2, select Roast, set temperature to 380ºF (193ºC), and set time to 12 minutes.
4. When cooking is complete, remove from the oven. Divide the mixture among four plates. Serve warm with a sprinkle of grated eggs and a drizzle of soy sauce.

249.Garlicky Veggie Bake

Servings: 3
Cooking Time: 25 Minutes
Ingredients:
- 3 turnips, sliced
- 1 large red onion, cut into rings
- 1 large zucchini, sliced
- Salt and black pepper to taste
- 2 cloves garlic, crushed
- 1 bay leaf, cut in 6 pieces
- 1 tbsp olive oil

Directions:
1. Place the turnips, onion, and zucchini in a bowl. Toss with olive oil, salt, and pepper.
2. Preheat Cuisinart on Air Fry function to 380 F. Place the veggies into a baking pan. Slip the bay leaves in the different parts of the slices and tuck the garlic cloves in between the slices. Cook for 15 minutes. Serve warm with as a side to a meat dish or salad.

250.Roasted Vegetable Mélange With Herbs

Servings:4
Cooking Time: 16 Minutes
Ingredients:
- 1 (8-ounce / 227-g) package sliced mushrooms
- 1 yellow summer squash, sliced
- 1 red bell pepper, sliced

- 3 cloves garlic, sliced
- 1 tablespoon olive oil
- ½ teaspoon dried basil
- ½ teaspoon dried thyme
- ½ teaspoon dried tarragon

Directions:
1. Toss the mushrooms, squash, and bell pepper with the garlic and olive oil in a large bowl until well coated. Mix in the basil, thyme, and tarragon and toss again.
2. Spread the vegetables evenly in the air fryer basket.
3. Put the air fryer basket on the baking pan and slide into Rack Position 2, select Roast, set temperature to 350ºF (180ºC), and set time to 16 minutes.
4. When cooking is complete, the vegetables should be fork-tender. Remove from the oven and cool for 5 minutes before serving.

251.Pumpkin French Cuisine Galette

Servings:x
Cooking Time:x
Ingredients:
- 2 or 3 green chilies finely chopped
- 1 ½ tbsp. lemon juice
- Salt and pepper to taste
- 2 tbsp. garam masala
- 1 cup sliced pumpkin
- 3 tsp. ginger finely chopped
- 1-2 tbsp. fresh coriander leaves

Directions:
1. Mix the ingredients in a clean bowl.
2. Mold this mixture into round and flat French Cuisine Galettes.
3. Wet the French Cuisine Galettes slightly with water.
4. Pre heat the Breville smart oven at 160 degrees Fahrenheit for 5 minutes. Place the French Cuisine Galettes in the fry basket and let them cook for another 25 minutes at the same temperature. Keep rolling them over to get a uniform cook. Serve either with mint sauce or ketchup.

252.Feta & Scallion Triangles

Servings:4
Cooking Time: 20 Minutes

Ingredients:
- 4 oz feta cheese, crumbled
- 2 sheets filo pastry
- 1 egg yolk, beaten
- 2 tbsp fresh parsley, finely chopped
- 1 scallion, finely chopped
- 2 tbsp olive oil
- Salt and black pepper to taste

Directions:
1. In a bowl, mix the yolk with the cheese, parsley, and scallion. Season with salt and black pepper. Cut each filo sheet in 3 strips. Put a teaspoon of the feta mixture on the bottom. Roll the strip in a spinning spiral way until the filling of the inside mixture is completely wrapped in a triangle.
2. Preheat Breville on Bake function to 360 F. Brush the surface of filo with olive oil. Place up to 5 triangles in the oven and press Start. Cook for 5 minutes. Lower the temperature to 330 F, cook for 3 more minutes or until golden brown.

253.Mushroom Pasta

Servings:x
Cooking Time:x
Ingredients:
- 2 cups sliced mushroom
- 2 tbsp. all-purpose flour
- 2 cups of milk
- 1 tsp. dried oregano
- ½ tsp. dried basil
- ½ tsp. dried parsley
- 1 cup pasta
- 1 ½ tbsp. olive oil
- A pinch of salt
- For tossing pasta:
- 1 ½ tbsp. olive oil
- Salt and pepper to taste
- ½ tsp. oregano
- ½ tsp. basil
- 2 tbsp. olive oil
- Salt and pepper to taste

Directions:
1. Boil the pasta and sieve it when done. You will need to toss the pasta in the ingredients mentioned above and set aside.

2. For the sauce, add the ingredients to a pan and bring the ingredients to a boil. Stir the sauce and continue to simmer to make a thicker sauce. Add the pasta to the sauce and transfer this into a glass bowl garnished with cheese.

3. Pre heat the Breville smart oven at 160 degrees for 5 minutes. Place the bowl in the basket and close it. Let it continue to cook at the same temperature for 10 minutes more. Keep stirring the pasta in between.

254. Mushroom French Cuisine Galette

Servings:x
Cooking Time:x
Ingredients:
- 2 or 3 green chilies finely chopped
- 1 ½ tbsp. lemon juice
- Salt and pepper to taste
- 2 tbsp. garam masala
- 2 cups sliced mushrooms
- 1 ½ cup coarsely crushed peanuts
- 3 tsp. ginger finely chopped
- 1-2 tbsp. fresh coriander leaves

Directions:
1. Mix the ingredients in a clean bowl.
2. Mold this mixture into round and flat French Cuisine Galettes.
3. Wet the French Cuisine Galettes slightly with water. Coat each French Cuisine Galette with the crushed peanuts.
4. Pre heat the Breville smart oven at 160 degrees Fahrenheit for 5 minutes. Place the French Cuisine Galettes in the fry basket and let them cook for another 25 minutes at the same temperature. Keep rolling them over to get a uniform cook. Serve either with mint sauce or ketchup.

255. Asparagus Spicy Lemon Kebab

Servings:x
Cooking Time:x
Ingredients:
- 3 tsp. lemon juice
- 2 tsp. garam masala
- 3 eggs
- 2 ½ tbsp. white sesame seeds
- 2 cups sliced asparagus

- 3 onions chopped
- 5 green chilies-roughly chopped
- 1 ½ tbsp. ginger paste
- 1 ½ tsp. garlic paste
- 1 ½ tsp. salt

Directions:
1. Grind the ingredients except for the egg and form a smooth paste. Coat the asparagus in the paste. Now, beat the eggs and add a little salt to it.
2. Dip the coated apricots in the egg mixture and then transfer to the sesame seeds and coat the asparagus. Place the vegetables on a stick.
3. Pre heat the Breville smart oven at 160 degrees Fahrenheit for around 5 minutes. Place the sticks in the basket and let them cook for another 25 minutes at the same temperature. Turn the sticks over in between the cooking process to get a uniform cook.

256. Black Gram French Cuisine Galette

Servings:x
Cooking Time:x
Ingredients:
- 2 or 3 green chilies finely chopped
- 1 ½ tbsp. lemon juice
- Salt and pepper to taste
- 2 cup black gram
- 2 medium potatoes boiled and mashed
- 1 ½ cup coarsely crushed peanuts
- 3 tsp. ginger finely chopped
- 1-2 tbsp. fresh coriander leaves

Directions:
1. Mix the ingredients in a clean bowl.
2. Mold this mixture into round and flat French Cuisine Galettes.
3. Wet the French Cuisine Galettes slightly with water.
4. Pre heat the Breville smart oven at 160 degrees Fahrenheit for 5 minutes. Place the French Cuisine Galettes in the fry basket and let them cook for another 25 minutes at the same temperature. Keep rolling them over to get a uniform cook. Serve either with mint sauce or ketchup.

257.Veg Momo's Recipe

Servings:x
Cooking Time:x
Ingredients:

- 2 tsp. ginger-garlic paste
- 2 tsp. soya sauce
- 2 tsp. vinegar
- 1 ½ cup all-purpose flour
- ½ tsp. salt or to taste
- 5 tbsp. water
- 2 cup carrots grated
- 2 cup cabbage grated
- 2 tbsp. oil

Directions:

1. Squeeze the dough and cover it with plastic wrap and set aside. Next, cook the ingredients for the filling and try to ensure that the vegetables are covered well with the sauce.
2. Roll the dough and cut it into a square. Place the filling in the center. Now, wrap the dough to cover the filling and pinch the edges together.
3. Pre heat the Breville smart oven at 200° F for 5 minutes. Place the gnocchi's in the fry basket and close it. Let them cook at the same temperature for another 20 minutes. Recommended sides are chili sauce or ketchup.

258.Cottage Cheese Gnocchi's

Servings:x
Cooking Time:x
Ingredients:

- 2 tsp. ginger-garlic paste
- 2 tsp. soya sauce
- 2 tsp. vinegar
- 1 ½ cup all-purpose flour
- ½ tsp. salt
- 5 tbsp. water
- 2 cups grated cottage cheese
- 2 tbsp. oil

Directions:

1. Squeeze the dough and cover it with plastic wrap and set aside. Next, cook the ingredients for the filling and try to ensure

that the cottage cheese is covered well with the sauce.
2. Roll the dough and place the filling in the center. Now, wrap the dough to cover the filling and pinch the edges together.
3. Pre heat the Breville smart oven at 200° F for 5 minutes. Place the gnocchi's in the fry basket and close it. Let them cook at the same temperature for another 20 minutes. Recommended sides are chili sauce or ketchup.

259.Potato Fries With Ketchup

Servings:2
Cooking Time: 20 Minutes
Ingredients:

- 2 potatoes
- 1 tbsp ketchup
- 2 tbsp olive oil
- Salt and black pepper to taste

Directions:

1. Use a spiralizer to spiralize the potatoes. In a bowl, mix olive oil, salt, and pepper. Drizzle the potatoes with the oil mixture. Place them in the basket and press Start. Cook for 15 minutes on AirFry function at 360 F. Serve with ketchup or mayonnaise.

260.Teriyaki Tofu

Servings:3
Cooking Time: 15 Minutes
Ingredients:

- Nonstick cooking spray
- 14 oz. firm or extra firm tofu, pressed & cut in 1-inch cubes
- ¼ cup cornstarch
- ½ tsp salt
- ½ tsp ginger
- ½ tsp white pepper
- 3 tbsp. olive oil
- 12 oz. bottle vegan teriyaki sauce

Directions:

1. Lightly spray baking pan with cooking spray.
2. In a shallow dish, combine cornstarch, salt, ginger, and pepper.
3. Heat oil in a large skillet over med-high heat.
4. Toss tofu cubes in cornstarch mixture then add to skillet. Cook 5 minutes, turning over

halfway through, until tofu is nicely seared. Transfer the tofu to the prepared baking pan.

5. Set oven to convection bake on 350°F for 15 minutes.
6. Pour all but ½ cup teriyaki sauce over tofu and stir to coat. After oven has preheated for 5 minutes, place the baking pan in position 2 and bake tofu 10 minutes.
7. Turn tofu over, spoon the sauce in the pan over it and bake another 10 minutes. Serve with reserved sauce for dipping.

- **Nutrition Info:** Calories 469, Total Fat 25g, Saturated Fat 4g, Total Carbs 33g, Net Carbs 30g, Protein 28g, Sugar 16g, Fiber 3g, Sodium 2424mg, Potassium 571mg, Phosphorus 428mg

261.Bottle Gourd Flat Cakes

Servings:x
Cooking Time:x
Ingredients:
- 2 or 3 green chilies finely chopped
- 1 ½ tbsp. lemon juice
- Salt and pepper to taste
- 2 tbsp. garam masala
- 2 cups sliced bottle gourd
- 3 tsp. ginger finely chopped
- 1-2 tbsp. fresh coriander leaves

Directions:
1. Mix the ingredients in a clean bowl and add water to it. Make sure that the paste is not too watery but is enough to apply on the bottle gourd slices. Pre heat the Breville smart oven at 160 degrees Fahrenheit for 5 minutes.
2. Place the French Cuisine Galettes in the fry basket and let them cook for another 25 minutes at the same temperature. Keep rolling them over to get a uniform cook. Serve either with mint sauce or ketchup.

262.Asparagus French Cuisine Galette

Servings:x
Cooking Time:x
Ingredients:
- 1 ½ tbsp. lemon juice
- Salt and pepper to taste
- 2 cups minced asparagus

- 3 tsp. ginger finely chopped
- 1-2 tbsp. fresh coriander leaves
- 2 or 3 green chilies finely chopped

Directions:
1. Mix the ingredients in a clean bowl.
2. Mold this mixture into round and flat French Cuisine Galettes.
3. Wet the French Cuisine Galettes slightly with water.
4. Pre heat the Breville smart oven at 160 degrees Fahrenheit for 5 minutes. Place the French Cuisine Galettes in the fry basket and let them cook for another 25 minutes at the same temperature. Keep rolling them over to get a uniform cook. Serve either with mint sauce or ketchup.

263.Cabbage Fritters(2)

Servings:x
Cooking Time:x
Ingredients:
- 1 ½ tsp. salt
- 3 tsp. lemon juice
- 2 tsp. garam masala
- 3 eggs
- 2 ½ tbsp. white sesame seeds
- 10 leaves cabbage
- 3 onions chopped
- 5 green chilies-roughly chopped
- 1 ½ tbsp. ginger paste
- 1 ½ tsp. garlic paste

Directions:
1. Grind the ingredients except for the egg and form a smooth paste. Coat the leaves in the paste. Now, beat the eggs and add a little salt to it.
2. Dip the coated leaves in the egg mixture and then transfer to the sesame seeds and coat the florets well. Place the vegetables on a stick.
3. Pre heat the Breville smart oven at 160 degrees Fahrenheit for around 5 minutes. Place the sticks in the basket and let them cook for another 25 minutes at the same temperature. Turn the sticks over in between the cooking process to get a uniform cook.

264.French Bean Toast

Servings:x
Cooking Time:x
Ingredients:
- 1 tsp. sugar for every 2 slices

- Crushed cornflakes
- 2 cups baked beans
- Bread slices (brown or white)
- 1 egg white for every 2 slices

Directions:
1. Put two slices together and cut them along the diagonal.
2. In a bowl, whisk the egg whites and add some sugar.
3. Dip the bread triangles into this mixture and then coat them with the crushed cornflakes.
4. Pre heat the Breville smart oven at 180° C for 4 minutes. Place the coated bread triangles in the fry basket and close it. Let them cook at the same temperature for another 20 minutes at least. Halfway through the process, turn the triangles over so that you get a uniform cook. Top with baked beans and serve.

265.Bean, Salsa, And Cheese Tacos

Servings:4
Cooking Time: 7 Minutes
Ingredients:
- 1 (15-ounce / 425-g) can black beans, drained and rinsed
- ½ cup prepared salsa
- 1½ teaspoons chili powder
- 4 ounces (113 g) grated Monterey Jack cheese
- 2 tablespoons minced onion
- 8 (6-inch) flour tortillas
- 2 tablespoons vegetable or extra-virgin olive oil
- Shredded lettuce, for serving

Directions:
1. In a medium bowl, add the beans, salsa and chili powder. Coarsely mash them with a potato masher. Fold in the cheese and onion and stir until combined.
2. Arrange the flour tortillas on a cutting board and spoon 2 to 3 tablespoons of the filling into each tortilla. Fold the tortillas over, pressing lightly to even out the filling. Brush the tacos on one side with half the olive oil and put them, oiled side down, in the air fryer basket. Brush the top side with the remaining olive oil.
3. Put the air fryer basket on the baking pan and slide into Rack Position 2, select Air Fry, set temperature to 400ºF (205ºC), and set time to 7 minutes.

4. Flip the tacos halfway through the cooking time.
5. Remove from the oven and allow to cool for 5 minutes. Serve with the shredded lettuce on the side.

266.Rosemary Butternut Squash Roast

Servings: 2
Cooking Time: 30 Minutes
Ingredients:
- 1 butternut squash
- 1 tbsp dried rosemary
- 2 tbsp maple syrup
- Salt to taste

Directions:
1. Place the squash on a cutting board and peel. Cut in half and remove the seeds and pulp. Slice into wedges and season with salt. Preheat Cuisinart on Air Fry function to 350 F. Spray the wedges with cooking spray and sprinkle with rosemary. Place the wedges in the basket without overlapping and fit in the baking tray. Cook for 20 minutes, flipping once halfway through. Serve with maple syrup and goat cheese.

267.Cheese And Mushroom Spicy Lemon Kebab

Servings:x
Cooking Time:x
Ingredients:
- 1-2 tbsp. all-purpose flour for coating purposes
- 1-2 tbsp. mint
- 1 cup molten cheese
- 1 onion that has been finely chopped
- ½ cup milk
- 2 cups sliced mushrooms
- 1-2 green chilies chopped finely
- ¼ tsp. red chili powder
- A pinch of salt to taste
- ½ tsp. dried mango powder
- ¼ tsp. black salt

Directions:
1. Take the mushroom slices and add the grated ginger and the cut green chilies. Grind this mixture until it becomes a thick paste.
2. Keep adding water as and when required. Now add the onions, mint, the breadcrumbs and all the various masalas required. Mix this well until you get a soft dough. Now take small balls of this mixture (about the

size of a lemon) and mold them into the shape of flat and round kebabs. Here is where the milk comes into play.

3. Pour a very small amount of milk onto each kebab to wet it. Now roll the kebab in the dry breadcrumbs. Pre heat the Breville smart oven for 5 minutes at 300 Fahrenheit. Take out the basket. Arrange the kebabs in the basket leaving gaps between them so that no two kebabs are touching each other. Keep the fryer at 340 Fahrenheit for around half an hour.

4. Half way through the cooking process, turn the kebabs over so that they can be cooked properly. Recommended sides for this dish are mint sauce, tomato ketchup or yoghurt sauce.

268.Stuffed Eggplant Baskets

Servings:x
Cooking Time:x
Ingredients:
- 1 tsp. cumin powder
- Salt and pepper to taste
- 3 tbsp. grated cheese
- 1 tsp. red chili flakes
- ½ tsp. oregano
- 6 eggplants
- ½ tsp. salt
- ½ tsp. pepper powder
- 1 medium onion finely chopped
- 1 green chili finely chopped
- 1 ½ tbsp. chopped coriander leaves
- 1 tsp. fenugreek
- 1 tsp. dried mango powder
- ½ tsp. basil
- ½ tsp. parsley

Directions:
1. Take all the ingredients under the heading "Filling" and mix them together in a bowl.
2. Remove the stem of the eggplant. Cut off the caps. Remove a little of the flesh as well. Sprinkle some salt and pepper on the inside of the capsicums.
3. Leave them aside for some time.
4. Now fill the eggplant with the filling prepared but leave a small space at the top. Sprinkle grated cheese and also add the seasoning.
5. Pre heat the Breville smart oven at 140 degrees Fahrenheit for 5 minutes. Put the capsicums in the fry basket and close it. Let them cook at the same temperature for

another 20 minutes. Turn them over in between to prevent over cooking.

269.Bitter Gourd Flat Cakes

Servings:x
Cooking Time:x
Ingredients:
- 2 or 3 green chilies finely chopped
- 1 ½ tbsp. lemon juice
- Salt and pepper to taste
- 2 tbsp. garam masala
- 2 cups sliced bitter gourd
- 3 tsp. ginger finely chopped
- 1-2 tbsp. fresh coriander leaves

Directions:
1. Mix the ingredients in a clean bowl and add water to it. Make sure that the paste is not too watery but is enough to apply on the bitter gourd slices.
2. Pre heat the Breville smart oven at 160 degrees Fahrenheit for 5 minutes. Place the French Cuisine Galettes in the fry basket and let them cook for another 25 minutes at the same temperature. Keep rolling them over to get a uniform cook. Serve either with mint sauce or ketchup.

270.Cauliflower Rice With Tofu & Peas

Servings: 4
Cooking Time: 30 Minutes
Ingredients:
- Tofu:
- ½ block tofu, crumbled
- ½ cup diced onion
- 2 tbsp soy sauce
- 1 tsp turmeric
- 1 cup diced carrot
- Cauliflower:
- 3 cups cauliflower rice
- 2 tbsp soy sauce
- ½ cup chopped broccoli
- 2 garlic cloves, minced
- 1 ½ tsp toasted sesame oil
- 1 tbsp minced ginger
- ½ cup frozen peas
- 1 tbsp rice vinegar

Directions:
1. Preheat Cuisinart on Air Fry function to 370 F. Combine all the tofu ingredients in a greased baking dish. Cook for 10 minutes.
2. Meanwhile, place all cauliflower ingredients in a large bowl and mix to combine. Stir the cauliflower mixture in the tofu baking dish

and return to the oven; cook for 12 minutes. Serve.

271.Vegetable Spicy Lemon Kebab

Servings:x
Cooking Time:x
Ingredients:
- 1 ½ tsp. salt
- 3 tsp. lemon juice
- 2 tsp. garam masala
- 4 tbsp. chopped coriander
- 3 tbsp. cream
- 3 tbsp. chopped capsicum
- 2 cups mixed vegetables
- 3 onions chopped
- 5 green chilies-roughly chopped
- 1 ½ tbsp. ginger paste
- 1 ½ tsp. garlic paste
- 3 eggs
- 2 ½ tbsp. white sesame seeds

Directions:
1. Grind the ingredients except for the egg and form a smooth paste. Coat the vegetables in the paste. Now, beat the eggs and add a little salt to it.
2. Dip the coated vegetables in the egg mixture and then transfer to the sesame seeds and coat the vegetables well. Place the vegetables on a stick.
3. Pre heat the Breville smart oven at 160 degrees Fahrenheit for around 5 minutes. Place the sticks in the basket and let them cook for another 25 minutes at the same temperature. Turn the sticks over in between the cooking process to get a uniform cook.

272.Baked Turnip And Zucchini

Servings:4
Cooking Time: 18 Minutes
Ingredients:
- 3 turnips, sliced
- 1 large zucchini, sliced
- 1 large red onion, cut into rings
- 2 cloves garlic, crushed
- 1 tablespoon olive oil
- Salt and black pepper, to taste

Directions:
1. Put the turnips, zucchini, red onion, and garlic in the baking pan. Drizzle the olive oil over the top and sprinkle with the salt and pepper.
2. Slide the baking pan into Rack Position 1, select Convection Bake, set temperature to 330ºF (166ºC), and set time to 18 minutes.
3. When cooking is complete, the vegetables should be tender. Remove from the oven and serve on a plate.

273.Buffalo Cauliflower

Servings: 2
Cooking Time: 15 Minutes
Ingredients:
- Cauliflower:
- 1 C. panko breadcrumbs
- 1 tsp. salt
- 4 C. cauliflower florets
- Buffalo Coating:
- ¼ C. Vegan Buffalo sauce
- ¼ C. melted vegan butter

Directions:
1. Preparing the Ingredients. Melt butter in microwave and whisk in buffalo sauce.
2. Dip each cauliflower floret into buffalo mixture, ensuring it gets coated well. Hold over a bowl till floret is done dripping.
3. Mix breadcrumbs with salt.
4. Air Frying. Dredge dipped florets into breadcrumbs and place into the air fryer oven. Set the temperature to 350°F, and set time to 15 minutes. When slightly browned, they are ready to eat!
5. Serve with your favorite keto dipping sauce!
- **Nutrition Info:** CALORIES: 194; FAT: 17G; PROTEIN:10G; SUGAR:

SNACKS AND DESSERTS RECIPES

274.Fried Pickles

Servings: 6
Cooking Time: 3 Minutes
Ingredients:

- Cold dill pickle slices, 36.
- Chopped fresh dill, 2 tbsps.
- Salt, 1 tsp.
- Divided cornstarch, 1 cup
- Ranch dressing
- Cayenne, ¼ tsp.
- Black pepper, 2 tsps.
- Almond meal, ½ cup
- Large egg, 1.
- Almond milk, ¾ cup
- Paprika, 2 tsps.
- Canola oil

Directions:

1. Whisk together cayenne, milk, and egg.
2. Spread half-cup cornstarch in a shallow dish.
3. Mix the remaining ½-cup cornstarch with almond meal, salt, pepper, dill, and paprika.
4. Dredge the pickle slices first through the cornstarch then dip them in an egg wash.
5. Coat them with almond meal mixture and shake off the excess.
6. Place them in the fryer basket and spray them with oil.
7. Return the basket to the fryer and air fry the pickles for 3 minutes at 3700 F working in batches as to not crowd the basket.
8. Serve warm.
- **Nutrition Info:** Calories: 138 Fat: 12.2 g Carbs: 5.8 g Protein: 4 g

275.Garlicky-lemon Zucchini

Servings:x
Cooking Time:x
Ingredients:

- Coarse salt and black pepper, to taste
- ½ tsp thyme, minced
- ½ lemon
- 4 small green zucchinis, any color, sliced about ¼-inch thick
- 1½ Tbsp extra virgin olive oil
- 1 Tbsp garlic, minced

Directions:

1. Heat Breville smart oven over medium-low heat. Add oil and let heat for 1 minute.
2. Sprinkle zucchini with salt and pepper.
3. Add to the pan in a single layer. When zucchini is nicely browned, flip
4. and brown on other side.
5. Add garlic and saute for 1 minute.
6. Sprinkle thyme and additional salt if necessary.
7. Remove from pan and squeeze lemon juice on zucchini.

276.Blueberry Pudding

Servings:x
Cooking Time:x
Ingredients:

- 2 tbsp. custard powder
- 3 tbsp. powdered sugar
- 3 tbsp. unsalted butter
- 1 cup blueberry juice
- 2 cups milk

Directions:

1. Boil the milk and the sugar in a pan and add the custard powder followed by the blueberry juice and stir till you get a thick mixture.
2. Preheat the fryer to 300 Fahrenheit for five minutes. Place the dish in the basket and reduce the temperature to 250 Fahrenheit. Cook for ten minutes and set aside to cool.

277.Green Chiles Nachos

Servings:6
Cooking Time: 10 Minutes
Ingredients:

- 8 ounces (227 g) tortilla chips
- 3 cups shredded Monterey Jack cheese, divided
- 2 (7-ounce / 198-g) cans chopped green chiles, drained
- 1 (8-ounce / 227-g) can tomato sauce
- ¼ teaspoon dried oregano
- ¼ teaspoon granulated garlic
- ¼ teaspoon freshly ground black pepper
- Pinch cinnamon
- Pinch cayenne pepper

Directions:

1. Arrange the tortilla chips close together in a single layer in the baking pan. Sprinkle 1½ cups of the cheese over the chips. Arrange the green chiles over the cheese as evenly as possible. Top with the remaining 1½ cups of the cheese.
2. Slide the baking pan into Rack Position 2, select Roast, set temperature to 375ºF (190ºC) and set time to 10 minutes.
3. Meanwhile, stir together the remaining ingredients in a bowl.
4. When cooking is complete, the cheese will be melted and starting to crisp around the edges of the pan. Remove from the oven. Drizzle the sauce over the nachos and serve warm.

278.Salsa Cheese Dip

Servings: 10
Cooking Time: 30 Minutes
Ingredients:

- 16 oz cream cheese, softened
- 3 cups cheddar cheese, shredded
- 1 cup sour cream
- 1/2 cup hot salsa

Directions:

1. Fit the Cuisinart oven with the rack in position
2. In a bowl, mix all ingredients until just combined and pour into the baking dish.
3. Set to bake at 350 F for 35 minutes. After 5 minutes place the baking dish in the preheated oven.
4. Serve and enjoy.
- **Nutrition Info:** Calories 348 Fat 31.9 g Carbohydrates 3.4 g Sugar 0.7 g Protein 12.8 g Cholesterol 96 mg

279.Yogurt Cake(1)

Servings: 12
Cooking Time: 15 Minutes
Ingredients:

- 6 eggs, whisked
- 8 oz. Greek yogurt
- 9 oz. coconut flour
- 4 tbsp. stevia
- 1 tsp. vanilla extract

- 1 tsp. baking powder

Directions:

1. Take a bowl and mix all the ingredients and whisk well.
2. Pour this into a cake pan that fits the air fryer lined with parchment paper.
3. Put the pan in the air fryer and cook at 330°F for 30 minutes
- **Nutrition Info:** Calories: 181; Fat: 13g; Fiber: 2g; Carbs: 4g; Protein: 5g

280.Flavorful Coconut Cake

Servings: 8
Cooking Time: 20 Minutes
Ingredients:

- 5 eggs, separated
- 1/2 cup erythritol
- 1/4 cup coconut milk
- 1/2 cup coconut flour
- 1/2 tsp baking powder
- 1/2 tsp vanilla
- 1/2 cup butter softened
- Pinch of salt

Directions:

1. Fit the Cuisinart oven with the rack in position
2. Grease cake pan with butter and set aside.
3. In a bowl, beat sweetener and butter until combined.
4. Add egg yolks, coconut milk, and vanilla and mix well.
5. Add baking powder, coconut flour, and salt and stir well.
6. In another bowl, beat egg whites until stiff peak forms.
7. Gently fold egg whites into the cake mixture.
8. Pour batter in a prepared cake pan.
9. Set to bake at 400 F for 25 minutes. After 5 minutes place the cake pan in the preheated oven.
10. Slice and serve.
- **Nutrition Info:** Calories 84 Fat 5.9 g Carbohydrates 4.2 g Sugar 0.6 g Protein 4 g Cholesterol 102 mg

281.Tasty Cauliflower Tots

Servings: 16
Cooking Time: 18 Minutes

Ingredients:

- 2 cups cauliflower, steamed and shredded
- 1 tbsp butter
- 1/2 cup parmesan cheese, shredded
- 1/4 tsp onion powder
- 1 large egg
- Pepper
- Salt

Directions:

1. Fit the Cuisinart oven with the rack in position
2. Add all ingredients to the bowl and mix well to combine.
3. Using a tablespoon make small tots from cauliflower mixture and arrange in baking pan.
4. Set to bake at 425 F for 23 minutes. After 5 minutes place the baking pan in the preheated oven.
5. Serve and enjoy.
- **Nutrition Info:** Calories 23 Fat 1.6 g Carbohydrates 0.8 g Sugar 0.3 g Protein 1.6 g Cholesterol 16 mg

282.Cream Caramel

Servings:x
Cooking Time:x

Ingredients:

- 3 tbsp. unsalted butter
- 4 tbsp. caramel
- 2 cups milk
- 2 cups custard powder
- 3 tbsp. powdered sugar

Directions:

1. Boil the milk and the sugar in a pan and add the custard powder and stir till you get a thick mixture.
2. Preheat the fryer to 300 Fahrenheit for five minutes. Place the dish in the basket and reduce the temperature to 250 Fahrenheit. Cook for ten minutes and set aside to cool.
3. Spread the caramel over the dish and serve warm.

283.Air Fryer Cabbage Chips

Servings: 6
Cooking Time: 25 Minutes

Ingredients:

- 1 large cabbage head, tear cabbage leaves into pieces
- 2 tbsp olive oil
- 1/4 cup parmesan cheese, grated
- Pepper
- Salt

Directions:

1. Fit the Cuisinart oven with the rack in position 2.
2. Add all ingredients into the large mixing bowl and toss well.
3. Add cabbage pieces to the air fryer basket then place an air fryer basket in the baking pan.
4. Place a baking pan on the oven rack. Set to air fry at 300 F for 25 minutes.
5. Serve and enjoy.
- **Nutrition Info:** Calories 104 Fat 5.7 g Carbohydrates 12.2 g Sugar 6.7 g Protein 3.9 g Cholesterol 3 mg

284.Choco-peanut Mug Cake

Servings: 1
Cooking Time: 20 Minutes

Ingredients:

- Softened butter, 1 tsp.
- Egg, 1.
- Peanut butter, 1 tbsp.
- Vanilla extract, ½ tsp.
- Erythritol, 2 tbsps.
- Unsweetened cocoa powder, 2 tbsps.
- Baking powder, ¼ tsp.
- Heavy cream, 1 tbsp.

Directions:

1. Preheat the air fryer for 5 minutes.
2. Combine all ingredients in a mixing bowl.
3. Pour into a greased mug.
4. Set in the air fryer basket and cook for 20 minutes at 400 ºF
- **Nutrition Info:** Calories: 293 Protein: 12.4g Fat: 23.3g Carbs: 8.5g

285.Egg Rolls

Servings:x
Cooking Time:x

Ingredients:

- 1 cup shredded Napa cabbage
- 2 tablespoons soy sauce

- 1 tablespoon oyster sauce
- 2 tablespoons cornstarch 1 tablespoon water
- 1 package egg roll wrappers
- 3 cups peanut oil
- ½ pound ground pork
- ½ pound ground shrimp
- 1 carrot, shredded
- 2 cloves garlic, minced
- 1 bunch green onions, finely chopped

Directions:
1. In a large skillet, brown ground pork until almost done. Add ground shrimp, carrot, and garlic; cook and stir for 4 to 6 minutes or until pork is cooked. Remove from heat, drain well, and add green onions, cabbage, soy sauce, and oyster sauce.
2. Combine cornstarch and water in a small bowl and blend well.
3. To form egg rolls, place one wrapper, point-side down, on work surface. Place 1 tablespoon filling 1 inch from corner. Brush all edges of the egg roll wrapper with cornstarch mixture. Fold point over filling, then fold in sides and roll up egg roll, using cornstarch mixture to seal as necessary.
4. At this point, egg rolls may be flash frozen, or you can flash freeze them after frying. Once frozen, pack, label, and freeze in rigid containers.
5. To reheat untried egg rolls: Fry the frozen rolls in peanut oil heated to 375ºF for 2 to 3 minutes, turning once, or until deep golden brown. To reheat fried egg rolls: Place frozen egg rolls on baking sheet. Bake at 375ºF for 8 to 10 minutes or until crisp and hot.

286.Vanilla Brownies With Chocolate Chips

Servings:2
Cooking Time: 25 Minutes
Ingredients:
- 1 whole egg, beaten
- ¼ cup chocolate chips
- 2 tbsp white sugar
- ⅓ cup flour
- 2 tbsp safflower oil

- 1 tsp vanilla
- ¼ cup cocoa powder

Directions:
1. Preheat Breville on Bake function to 320 F. In a bowl, mix the beaten egg, sugar, oil, and vanilla. In another bowl, mix cocoa powder and flour. Add in the egg mixture and stir until incorporated.
2. Pour the mixture into a greased baking pan and sprinkle chocolate chips on top. Press Start. Bake for 20 minutes. Chill and cut into squares to serve.

287.Authentic Raisin Apple Treat

Servings: 4
Cooking Time: 15 Minutes
Ingredients:
- 4 apples, cored
- 1 ½ oz almonds
- ¾ oz raisins
- 2 tbsp sugar

Directions:
1. Preheat Cuisinart on Bake function to 360 F. In a bowl, mix sugar, almonds, and raisins. Blend the mixture using a hand mixer. Fill cored apples with the almond mixture. Place the apples in a baking tray and cook for 10 minutes. Serve with a sprinkle of powdered sugar.

288.Easy Lemon Cheesecake

Servings: 8
Cooking Time: 55 Minutes
Ingredients:
- 4 eggs
- 2 tbsp swerve
- 1 fresh lemon juice
- 18 oz ricotta cheese
- 1 fresh lemon zest

Directions:
1. Fit the Cuisinart oven with the rack in position
2. In a large bowl, beat ricotta cheese until smooth.
3. Add egg one by one and whisk well.
4. Add lemon juice, lemon zest, and swerve and mix well.
5. Transfer mixture into the greased cake pan.

6. Set to bake at 350 F for 60 minutes. After 5 minutes place the cake pan in the preheated oven.
7. Slice and serve.
- **Nutrition Info:** Calories 122 Fat 7.3 g Carbohydrates 4.2 g Sugar 0.5 g Protein 10.1 g Cholesterol 102 mg

289.Keto Mixed Berry Crumble Pots

Servings: 6
Cooking Time: 15 Minutes
Ingredients:
- 2 ounces unsweetened mixed berries
- 1/2 cup granulated swerve
- 2 tablespoons golden flaxseed meal
- 1/4 teaspoon ground star anise
- 1/2 teaspoon ground cinnamon
- 1 teaspoon xanthan gum
- 2/3 cup almond flour
- 1 cup powdered swerve
- 1/2 teaspoon baking powder
- 1/3 cup unsweetened coconut, finely shredded
- 1/2 stick butter, cut into small pieces

Directions:
1. Toss the mixed berries with the granulated swerve, golden flaxseed meal, star anise, cinnamon, and xanthan gum. Divide between six custard cups coated with cooking spray.
2. In a mixing dish, thoroughly combine the remaining ingredients. Sprinkle over the berry mixture.
3. Bake in the preheated Air Fryer at 330 degrees F for 35 minutes. Work in batches if needed.
- **Nutrition Info:** 155 Calories; 13g Fat; 1g Carbs; 1g Protein; 8g Sugars; 6g Fiber

290.Apple Treat With Raisins

Servings:4
Cooking Time: 15 Minutes
Ingredients:
- 4 apples, cored
- 1 ½ oz almonds
- ¾ oz raisins
- 2 tbsp sugar

Directions:

1. Preheat Breville on Bake function to 360 F. In a bowl, mix sugar, almonds, and raisins and blend the mixture using a hand mixer. Fill cored apples with the almond mixture. Place the prepared apples in the basket and press Start. Bake for 10 minutes. Serve with powdered sugar.

291.Cranberry Pancakes

Servings:x
Cooking Time:x
Ingredients:
- 2 tsp. dried parsley
- Salt and Pepper to taste
- 3 tbsp. Butter
- 2 cups minced cranberry
- 1 ½ cups almond flour
- 3 eggs
- 2 tsp. dried basil

Directions:
1. Preheat the air fryer to 250 Fahrenheit.
2. In a small bowl, mix the ingredients together. Ensure that the mixture is smooth and well balanced.
3. Take a pancake mold and grease it with butter. Add the batter to the mold and place it in the air fryer basket. Cook till both the sides of the pancake have browned on both sides and serve with maple syrup.

292.Air Fryer Radish Chips

Servings: 12
Cooking Time: 15 Minutes
Ingredients:
- 1 lb radish, wash and slice into chips
- 1/4 tsp pepper
- 2 tbsp olive oil
- 1 tsp salt

Directions:
1. Fit the Cuisinart oven with the rack in position 2.
2. Add all ingredients into the large bowl and toss well.
3. Add radish slices to the air fryer basket then place an air fryer basket in baking pan.
4. Place a baking pan on the oven rack. Set to air fry at 375 F for 15 minutes.
5. Serve and enjoy.

- **Nutrition Info:** Calories 26 Fat 2.4 g Carbohydrates 1.3 g Sugar 0.7 g Protein 0.3 g Cholesterol 0 mg

293.Spicy Cauliflower Florets

Servings: 4
Cooking Time: 15 Minutes
Ingredients:

- 1 medium cauliflower head, cut into florets
- 1/2 tsp old bay seasoning
- 1/4 tsp paprika
- 1/4 tsp cayenne
- 1/4 tsp chili powder
- 1 tbsp garlic, minced
- 3 tbsp olive oil
- Pepper
- Salt

Directions:

1. Fit the Cuisinart oven with the rack in position 2.
2. In a bowl, toss cauliflower with remaining ingredients.
3. Add cauliflower florets in air fryer basket then place air fryer basket in baking pan.
4. Place a baking pan on the oven rack. Set to air fry at 400 F for 15 minutes.
5. Serve and enjoy.
- **Nutrition Info:** Calories 130 Fat 10.7 g Carbohydrates 8.6 g Sugar 3.5 g Protein 3 g Cholesterol 0 mg

294.Three Berry Crumble

Servings:x
Cooking Time:x
Ingredients:

- ¾ cup brown sugar
- ¾ cup old fashioned oats
- ½ cup chopped almonds
- 1 tsp cinnamon
- 6 cups of fresh mixed berries (blueberries, raspberries), washed and dried
- ¼ cup sugar
- ¼ cup flour
- 1 Tbsp lemon juice
- ¾ cup flour
- 1 stick cold butter, cut into cubes

Directions:

1. Preheat oven to 375°F.
2. Lightly toss the berries, sugar, flour and lemon juice inside your Breville smart oven.
3. In a bowl, mix the flour, brown sugar, oats, almonds and cinnamon.
4. Incorporate cold butter with your fingertips into the oat mixture until small clumps form.
5. Pour topping onto fruit and bake for 45 minutes to 1 hour, until bubbles form and top appears browned and crispy.
6. Serve with vanilla ice cream right out of Breville smart oven.

295.Nutty Parmesan Homemade Fried Sticks

Servings:x
Cooking Time:x
Ingredients:

- ½ cup grated Parmesan cheese
- Teas
- 1 package frozen puff pastry sheets, thawed
- ½ cup ground almonds

Directions:

1. Preheat oven to 375ºF. In a small bowl, combine almonds, cheese, and pepper; blend well. Sprinkle half of this mixture over work surface and cover with one sheet puff pastry. Using a rolling pin, gently press pastry into cheese mixture. Turn pastry over and press cheese mixture into other side of pastry. Repeat with other half of cheese mixture and second sheet of puff pastry.
2. Using pastry cutter or sharp knife, cut pastry into ½-inch strips. Place on parchment paper- or foil-lined baking sheets, twisting each strip several times. Bake at 375ºF for 10 to 15 minutes or until browned and crisp, being careful not to burn sticks. Remove from baking sheet and cool completely on wire racks. Pack carefully into rigid containers, separating layers with waxed paper. Label containers and freeze.
3. To thaw and reheat: Thaw sticks at room temperature and serve, or carefully place frozen sticks on baking sheet and bake at 350ºF for 4 to 5 minutes or until hotpot cayenne pepper

296.Plum Cream(2)

Servings: 4
Cooking Time: 15 Minutes
Ingredients:

- 1 lb. plums, pitted and chopped.
- 1 ½ cups heavy cream
- ¼ cup swerve
- 1 tbsp. lemon juice

Directions:

1. Take a bowl and mix all the ingredients and whisk really well.
2. Divide this into 4 ramekins, put them in the air fryer and cook at 340°F for 20 minutes. Serve cold
- **Nutrition Info:** Calories: 171; Fat: 4g; Fiber: 2g; Carbs: 4g; Protein: 4g

297.Banana Pudding

Servings:x
Cooking Time:x
Ingredients:

- 3 tbsp. unsalted butter
- 3 tbsp. chopped mixed nuts
- 1 cup banana juice
- 2 cups milk
- 2 tbsp. custard powder
- 3 tbsp. powdered sugar

Directions:

1. Boil the milk and the sugar in a pan and add the custard powder followed by the banana juice and stir till you get a thick mixture.
2. Preheat the fryer to 300 Fahrenheit for five minutes. Place the dish in the basket and reduce the temperature to 250 Fahrenheit. Cook for ten minutes and set aside to cool. Garnish with nuts.

298.Air Fried Lemon-pepper Wings

Servings:10
Cooking Time: 24 Minutes
Ingredients:

- 2 pounds (907 g) chicken wings
- 4½ teaspoons salt-free lemon pepper seasoning
- 1½ teaspoons baking powder
- 1½ teaspoons kosher salt

Directions:

1. In a large bowl, toss together all the ingredients until well coated. Place the wings in the air fryer basket, making sure they don't crowd each other too much.
2. Put the air fryer basket on the baking pan and slide into Rack Position 2, select Air Fry, set temperature to 375ºF (190ºC) and set time to 24 minutes.
3. After 12 minutes, remove from the oven. Use tongs to turn the wings over. Return to the oven to continue cooking.
4. When cooking is complete, the wings should be dark golden brown and a bit charred in places. Remove from the oven and let rest for 5 minutes before serving.

299.Rosemary Roasted Almonds

Servings: 12
Cooking Time: 20 Minutes
Ingredients:

- 2 1/2 cups almonds
- 1 tbsp fresh rosemary, chopped
- 1 tbsp olive oil
- 2 ½ tbsp maple syrup
- 1/4 tsp cayenne
- 1/4 tsp ground coriander
- 1/4 tsp cumin
- 1/4 tsp chili powder
- Pinch of salt

Directions:

1. Fit the Cuisinart oven with the rack in position
2. Spray a baking tray with cooking spray and set aside.
3. In a mixing bowl, whisk together oil, cayenne, coriander, cumin, chili powder, rosemary, maple syrup, and salt.
4. Add almond and stir to coat.
5. Spread almonds in baking pan.
6. Set to bake at 325 F for 20 minutes. After 5 minutes place the baking pan in the preheated oven.
7. Serve and enjoy.
- **Nutrition Info:** Calories 137 Fat 11.2 g Carbohydrates 7.3 g Sugar 3.3 g Protein 4.2 g Cholesterol 0 mg

300.Apple Cake

Servings: 12
Cooking Time: 45 Minutes
Ingredients:

- 2 cups apples, peeled and chopped
- 1/4 cup sugar
- 1/4 cup butter, melted
- 12 oz apple juice
- 3 cups all-purpose flour
- 3 tsp baking powder
- 1 1/2 tbsp ground cinnamon
- 1 tsp Salt

Directions:

1. Fit the Cuisinart oven with the rack in position
2. In a large bowl, mix together flour, salt, sugar, cinnamon, and baking powder.
3. Add melted butter and apple juice and mix until well combined.
4. Add apples and fold well.
5. Pour batter into the greased baking dish.
6. Set to bake at 350 F for 45 minutes. After 5 minutes place the baking dish in the preheated oven.
7. Serve and enjoy.

- **Nutrition Info:** Calories 200 Fat 4 g Carbohydrates 38 g Sugar 11 g Protein 3 g Cholesterol 10 mg

CPSIA information can be obtained
at www.ICGtesting.com
Printed in the USA
LVHW060814110121
676184LV00015B/620